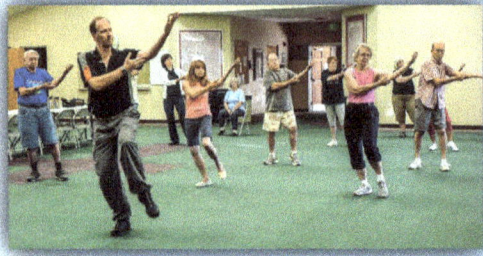
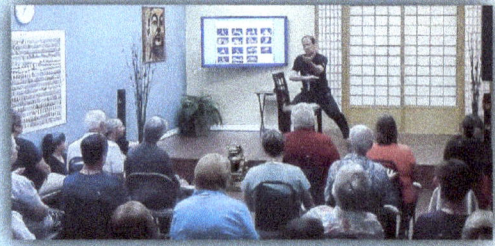
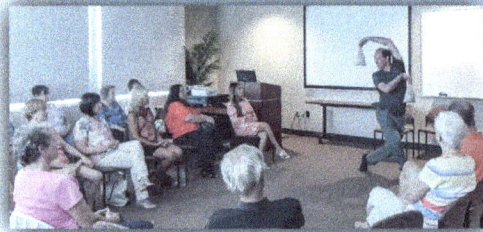
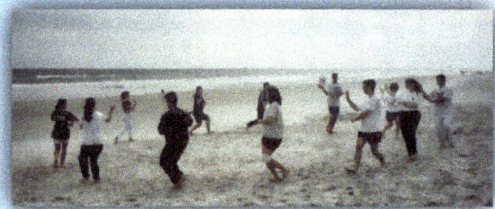
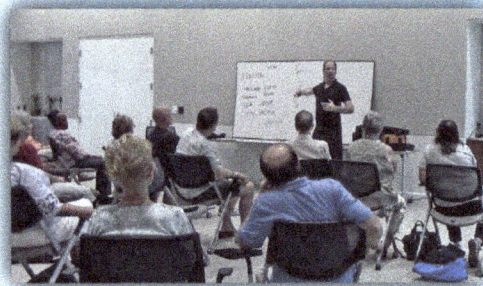
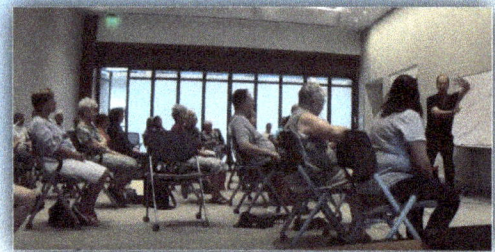
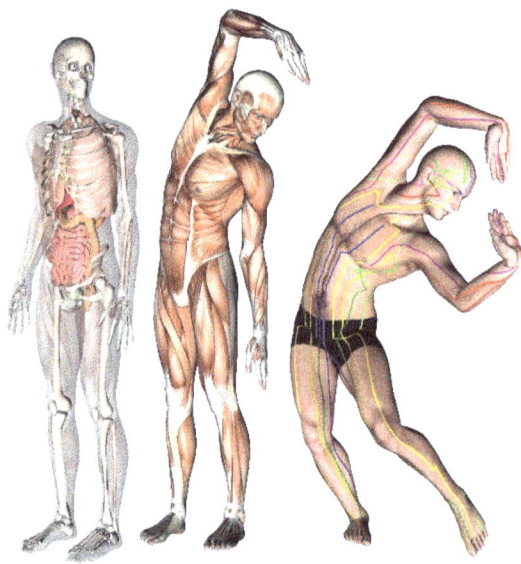

# Foreword

I am excited to present *The Wellness Chronicles*, a culmination of insights gathered from my many past years of writing on holistic health. This book distills key concepts from hundreds of my articles, offering a practical and thought-provoking guide to achieving well-being through a balanced approach to life.

In today's fast-paced world, where stress and pharmaceutical dependency often overshadow self-care and preventative health, *The Wellness Chronicles* serves as a beacon for those seeking a deeper understanding of the mind-body-spirit connection. It explores a broad spectrum of topics, including nutrition, physiology, healthcare modalities, meditation, psychology, and philosophy, all with an underlying focus on empowering individuals to take charge of their own well-being.

Readers will discover time-honored healing traditions such as Traditional Chinese Medicine (TCM) and Ayurveda, alongside modern holistic approaches that emphasize balance and harmony. This book encourages self-awareness and practical application, addressing injuries and ailments through natural, non-pharmaceutical solutions while advocating for movement, breathwork, and mindfulness as essential tools for health.

Beyond physical well-being, *The Wellness Chronicles* delves into the intricate connections between mind and body—how emotions, thought patterns, and beliefs influence our nervous system, stress responses, and overall vitality. These principles are supported by both ancient wisdom and contemporary insights, illustrating the profound interplay between psychology, philosophy, and personal transformation.

As a visual complement to these insights, I have included many of my original graphics throughout the book. These illustrations highlight self-regulation techniques, eclectic exercises, and Eastern methodologies, demonstrating how the intentional control of breath (wind), circulation (water), and mental focus can cultivate resilience, restore balance, and increase vitality (fire), a reflection of the Taoist concept that *"wind and water create fire."*

*The Wellness Chronicles* is more than a guide. It is an invitation to reflect, explore, and apply holistic principles in everyday life. My hope is that this book serves as both a resource and an inspiration, encouraging deeper inquiry into the art of living well.

Thank you for your engagement with this work. I am eager to share this journey with you and contribute to the collective pursuit of enduring health, happiness, and fulfillment.

Sincerely,

*Jim Moltzan*

## Why I Share, What I Have Learned

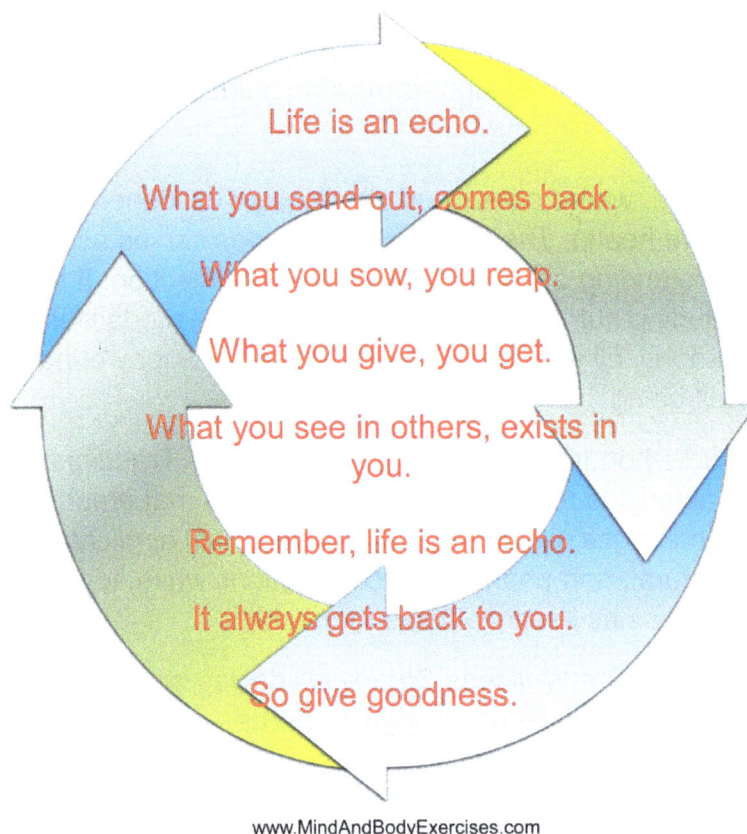

Life is an echo.

What you send out, comes back.

What you sow, you reap.

What you give, you get.

What you see in others, exists in you.

Remember, life is an echo.

It always gets back to you.

So give goodness.

www.MindAndBodyExercises.com

I made my commitment many years ago to learn, study, practice and teach fitness and well-being. My education came from martial arts and various other Eastern methods rooted in Traditional Chinese Medicine (TCM). I started when I was 16 years old and have never stopped since; 61 now.

I have written journals, produced educational graphics and co-authored a book in addition to many that I have self-authored. I blog often with a WordPress site, writing about the anatomical, physiological and mental benefits of mind and body training. Years back I started recording my classes and lectures, knowing that somewhere down the line, all of this information would be valuable to those who need and desire it.

My YouTube channel has almost 300 videos of FREE classes and other education videos. The goal all along has been to raise the awareness that Tai chi (a martial art), qigong (yoga at its root) and many other Eastern wellness methods, have proven the test of time for maintaining well-being. No gym, no mat, no membership, no special clothes or equipment. Just the individual and their engagement.

Weak or injured knees, back issues (strains & sciatica), stress & anxiety, asthma, arthritis, balance, poor posture - the list is endless. These are all issues that can be improved or overcome by those serious about learning about the mind, body & spirit connection.

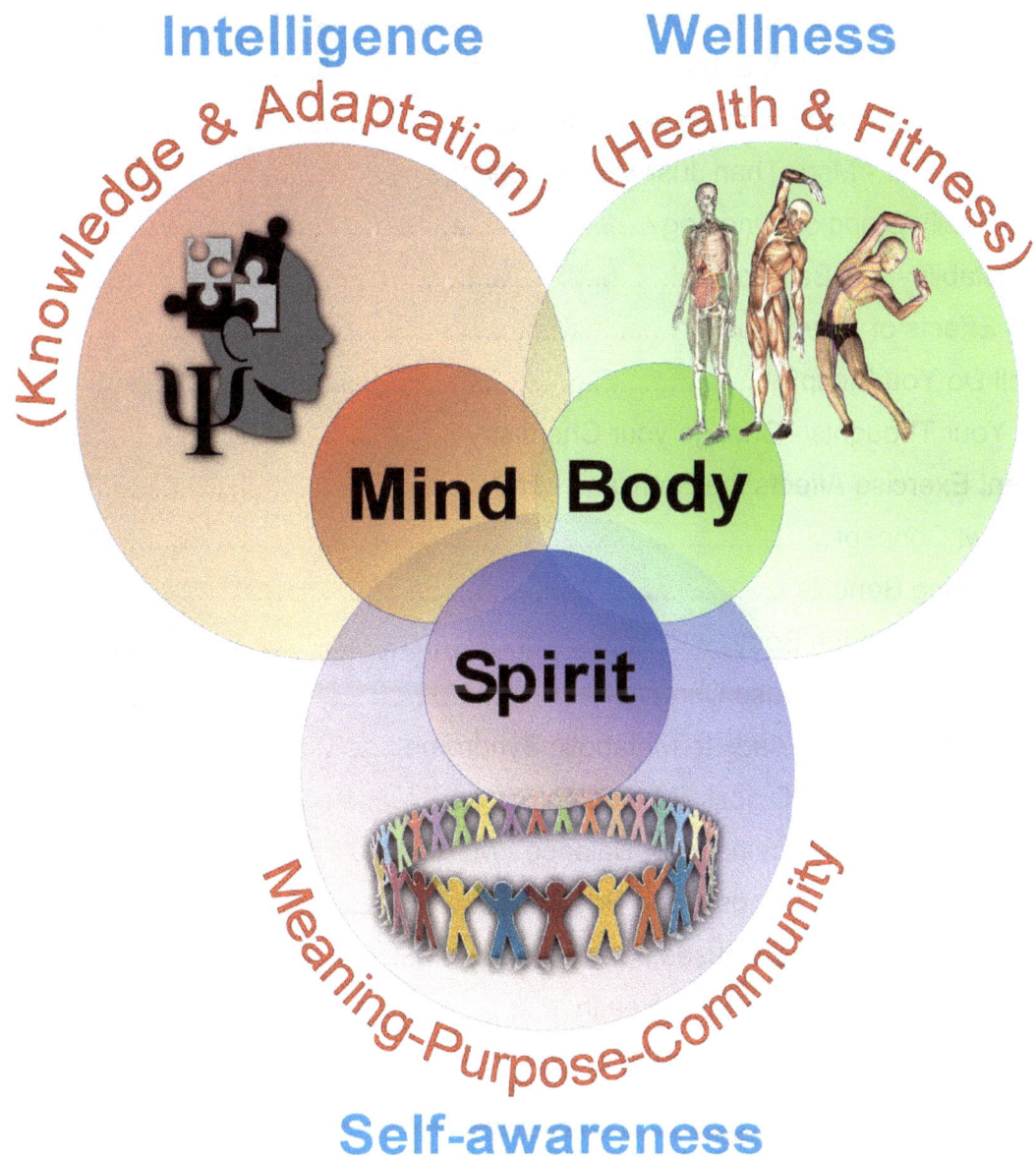

Intelligence  Wellness

(Knowledge & Adaptation)  (Health & Fitness)

Mind  Body

Spirit

Meaning-Purpose-Community

Self-awareness

*We are the architect of our own health, happiness, destiny, or fate.*

# Table of Contents

Basic Shoulder Anatomy & Exercises to Increase Strength & Range of Motion

Often people experience shoulder issues such as injuries, weaknesses and poor range of motion. Some exercise with running, stretching and weight training with little or no knowledge of how they should proceed with improving their particular issues. By practicing low impact exercises that focus more on strength and flexibility of the shoulder joint and its components, one can improve many issues without taking more drastic options such as pain medicines or surgery.

# Basic Shoulder Anatomy

**The human shoulder joint is a complex structure consisting of 4 joints and 3 bones:**

1) Glenohumeral joint
2) Acromioclavicular joint
3) Sternoclavicular joint
4) Scapulothoracic joint

1) clavicle (collar bone)
2) scapula (shoulder blade)
3) humerus, upper arm bone

This structure of joints and bones allows your shoulder to move in various directions. Each movement has a different degree of mobility. The ability of the shoulders to move in a normal range depends on the health of your:

1) muscles
2) ligaments
3) bones
4) individual joints

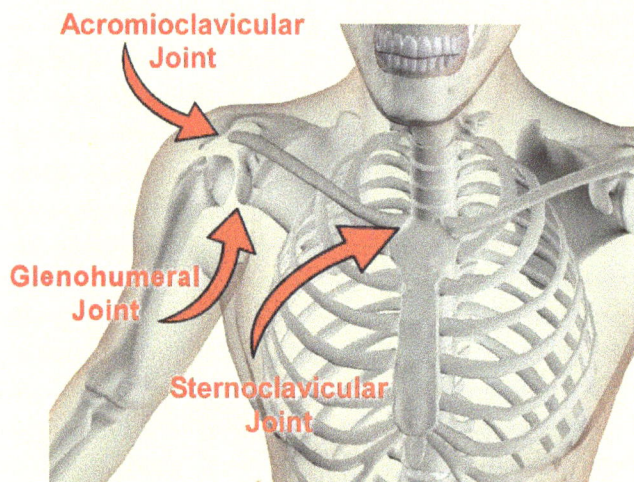

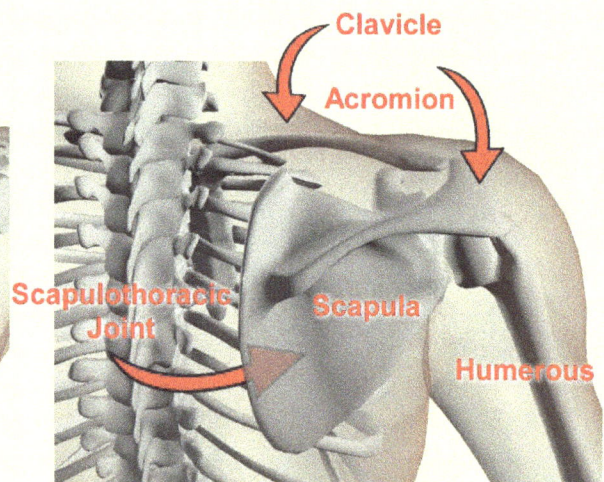

**Acromioclavicular Joint**

**Glenohumeral Joint**

**Sternoclavicular Joint**

**Clavicle**

**Acromion**

**Scapulothoracic Joint**

**Scapula**

**Humerous**

**www.MindandBodyExercises.com**   Ⓒ Copyright 2020 - CAD Graphics, Inc.

Additionally, having some knowledge of how the shoulder joint is composed and the natural range of motion can help the individual to have a better understanding of what the exercises are doing and set better goals and expectations.

# 8 Directions of Mobility

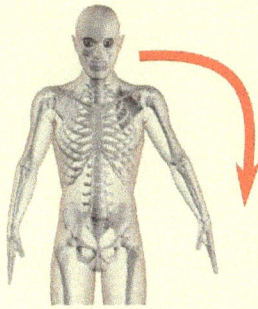
**Adduction**

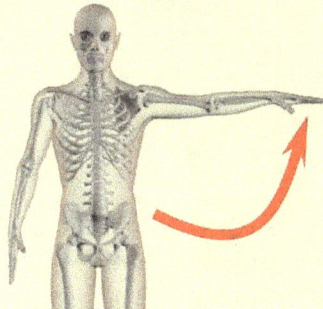
**Abduction**

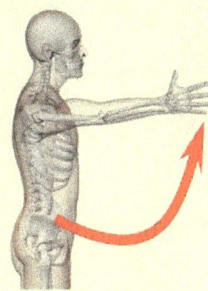
**Flexion**

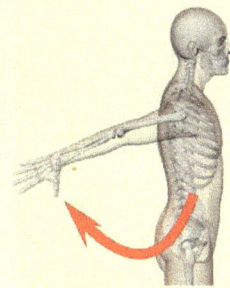
**Extension**

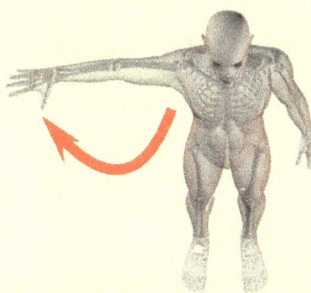
**Horizontal Abduction**

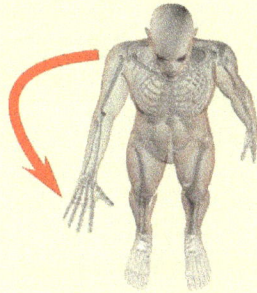
**Horizontal Adduction**

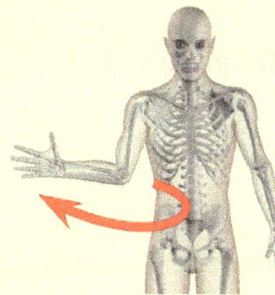
**Lateral Rotation**

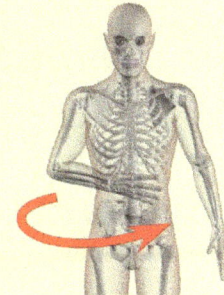
**Medial Rotation**

www.MindandBodyExercises.com     © Copyright 2020 - CAD Graphics, Inc.

## Shoulder Exercises Using Dynamic Tension and/or Light Weights

The following exercises are fairly simple and can be performed with or without dumbbells. The main goal is to increase strength within the natural range of motion in the neck, shoulders, arms, spine, hips, thighs and ankles. Light weights can help to tone muscles as well as provide increased strength in less used muscle groups. Weight training, even with lighter weights, has been known to help prevent osteoporosis. These exercises take up very little space and a few minutes of time to gain benefits. There should be a deep inhale at the start of each exercise, lasting about 4 seconds, followed by a deep 4 second exhalation as finishing the exercise. The muscles should remain relaxed while moving and flexed at the end position.

## Exercise #1

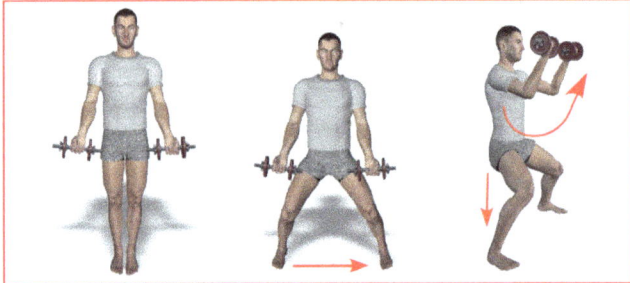

Start with dumbbells at thighs, palms forward. Step feet to double shoulder width apart. Drop the hips while keeping foot, knee and thigh within the same vertical plane. Raise hands up to eye-level by bending slowly from the elbows.

**www.MindandBodyExercises.com**

## Exercise #2

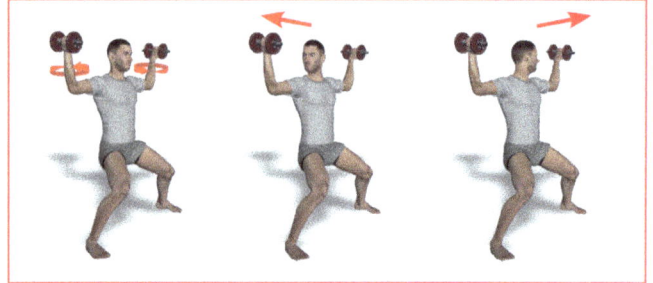

From previous position, rotate both wrists outward as turning head as far as possible to the right and then to the left. Again, drop the hips while keeping foot, knee and thigh within the same vertical plane. Exhale deeply as sinking the hips.

## Exercise #3

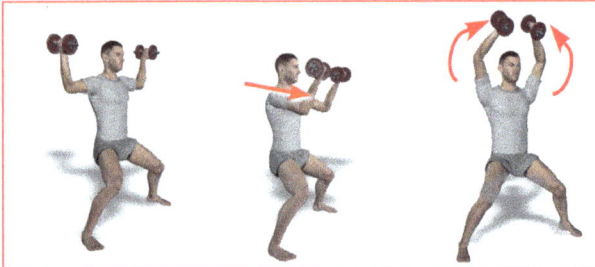

From previous position, rotate both wrists in toward your centerline. Rotate wrist outward and upward as raising both arms above the head. Exhale deeply as sinking the hips.

**www.MindandBodyExercises.com**

## Exercise #4

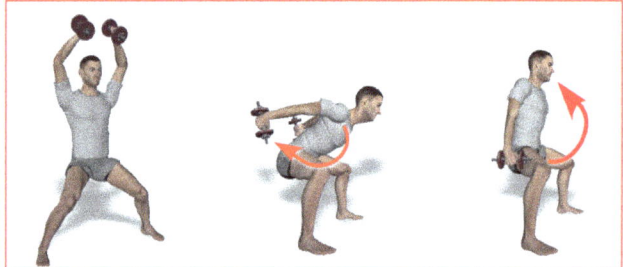

From previous position, bend forward at the waist as slowly raise arms behind the body and level with the ground. Exhale deeply as sinking the hips. Slowly drops arms to hips as the spine straightens upright.

Here are a few somewhat more advanced exercises.  Try and use a bean bag or a sock filled with small pebbles. Then you can adjust the amount of weight as you gain more strength in your muscles and joints. Lighter weight is always better than too heavy, which often can lead to more pain or discomfort.

**Exercise #5**

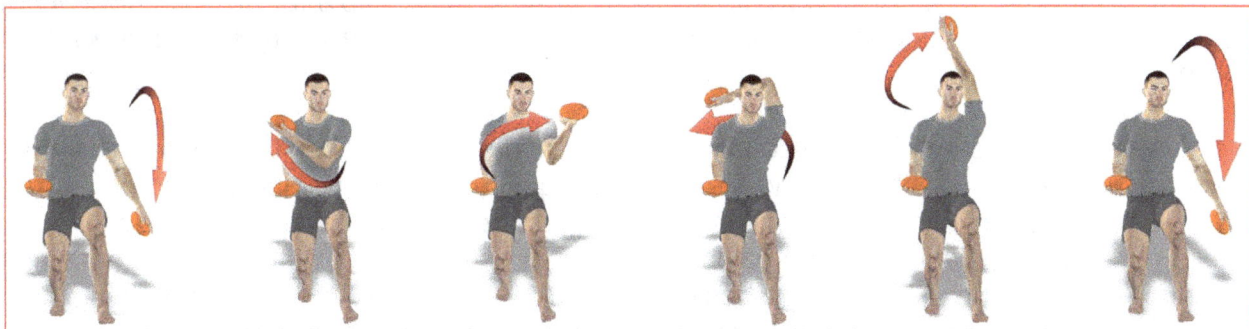

**Exercise #6**

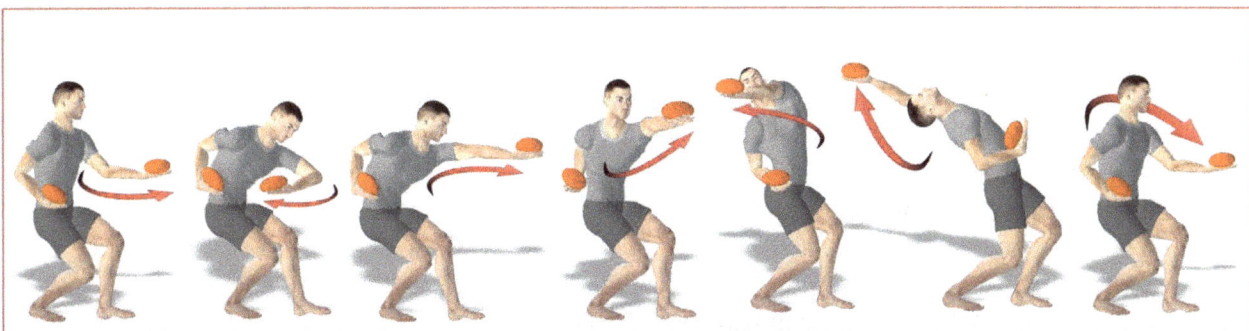

**www.MindandBodyExercises.com**     ⓒ Copyright 2020 - CAD Graphics, Inc.

4

## Blood Shunting (redirecting of the blood flow)

Shunting or accommodation means redirecting or diverting, specifically blood, to where it is needed most. Blood goes mostly to the skeletal muscles when exercising. When resting, blood goes mostly to the internal organs. This is why you can get stomach cramps when exercising soon after eating.

Why is this important to know? As we try to become more responsible for our own healthcare, it is extremely helpful to understand how your body works. **It is your body and your well-being!**

When you take your car in for service for maintenance or repairs, doesn't it help to know the difference between an oil change and a blown head gasket? If your home needs repairs, don't you try to become knowledgeable about the costs before you get a new roof or air conditioner? Your health is far more valuable than your car, house or other material assets. It pays off in the long run to learn some basics facts about your body, anatomy and physiology before becoming ill or injured. Gaining this knowledge while in the emergency room or doctor's office is usually not a fun way to learn about your health.

**During Normal Rest:**

- 15-20% of cardiac output is directed to skeletal muscles
- the liver receives 25%
- the kidneys receive 20%
- Blood is mostly in the organs

**During Exercise:**
During physical activity, blood flow is redirected to oxygen starved muscles and away from inactive organs. As body heat increases, some blood flow is redirected to the skin to help maintain internal body temperature.

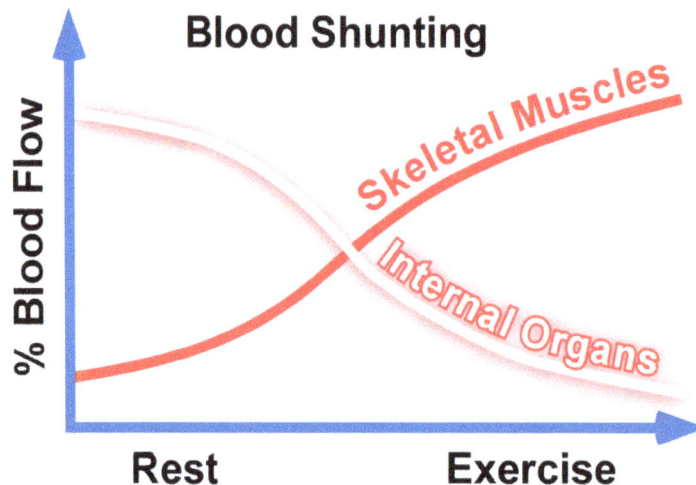

**During Eating:**
Blood flow is shunted to the engaged digestive system and decreased from the skeletal muscles. This is why stomach cramps can occur if exercising too soon after eating.

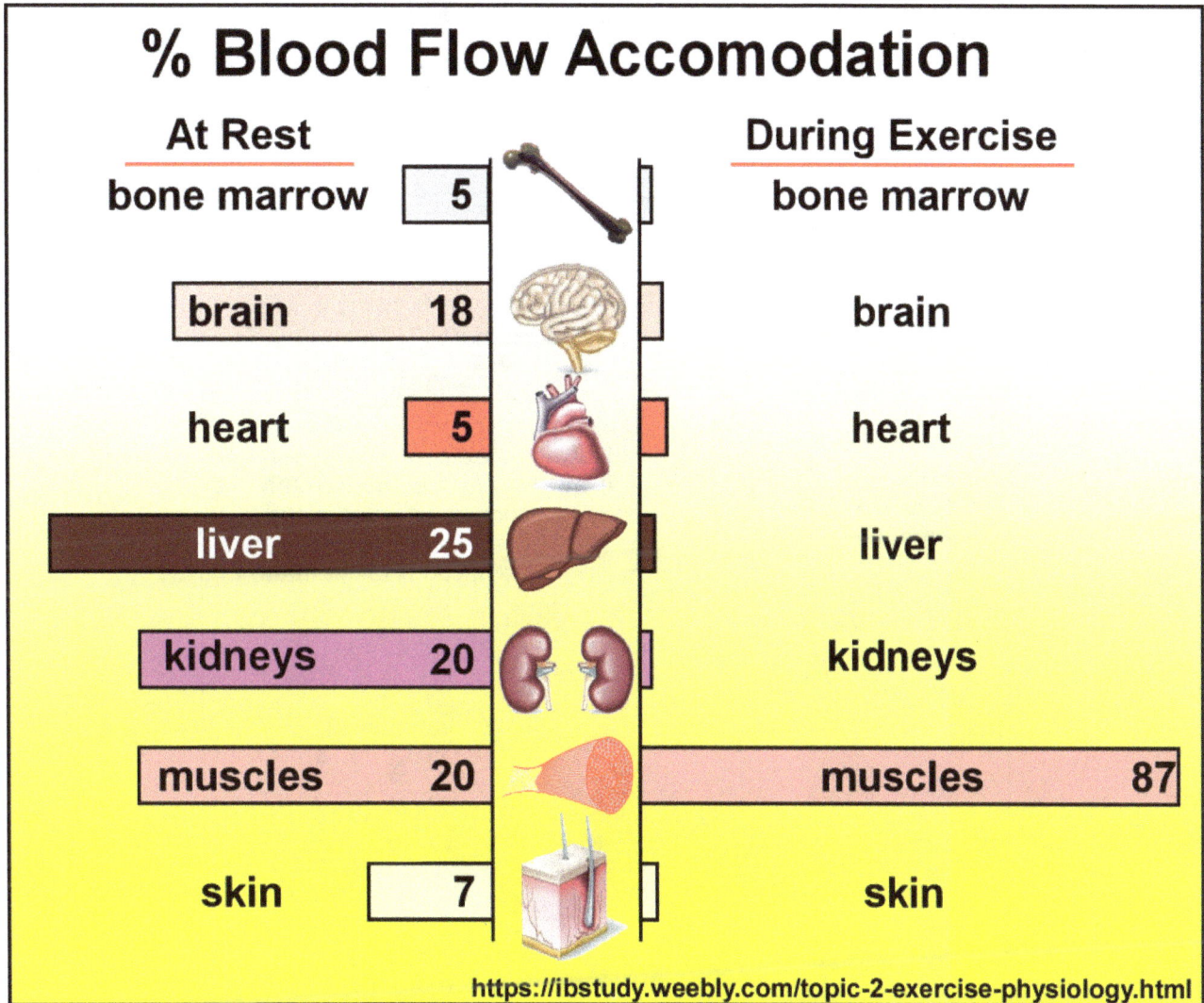

# % Blood Flow Accomodation

| At Rest | | During Exercise |
|---|---|---|
| bone marrow | 5 | bone marrow |
| brain | 18 | brain |
| heart | 5 | heart |
| liver | 25 | liver |
| kidneys | 20 | kidneys |
| muscles | 20 | muscles 87 |
| skin | 7 | skin |

https://ibstudy.weebly.com/topic-2-exercise-physiology.html

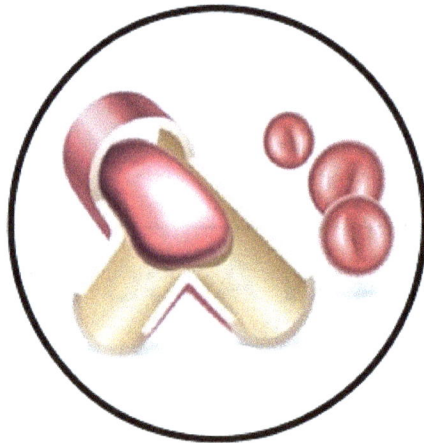

## Shunting or Accommodation

Means to redirect or divert, specifically blood to where it is needed most.

### During Normal Rest:

- 15-20% of cardiac output is directed to skeletal muscles
- the liver receives 25%
- the kidneys receive 20%

**Blood is mostly in the organs**

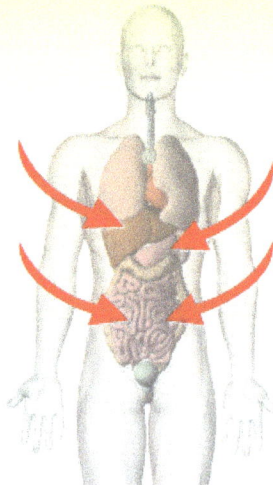

### During Exercise:

During physical activity, blood flow is redirected to oxygen starved muscles and away from inactive organs. As body heat increases, some blood flow is redirected to the skin to help maintain internal body temperature.

**Blood is mostly in the muscles**

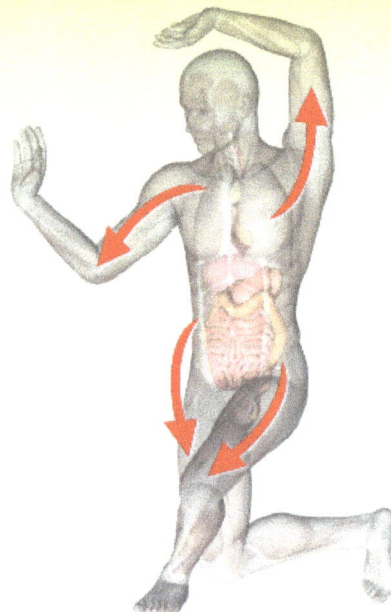

### During Eating:

Blood flow is shunted to the engaged digestive system, and decreased from the skeletal muscles. This is why stomach cramps can occur if exercising too soon after eating.

Learning how to regulate the breath is truly one of the key components to maintaining good health and well-being. Most people do not regulate their breath or even think about it, until a health issue presents itself.

Breathing shallow helps the body to produce cortisol and adrenaline. Breathing deeper helps the body to produce dopamine, oxytocin, serotonin and endorphins.

Controlling how you breathe can affect your emotions.

Emotions cause the brain to adjust and affect the body's blood chemistry.

The blood chemistry directly affects the internal organs and consequently all of the bodily systems and functions.

Watch my online instructions to get a better understanding of how and why to breathe deeper:

https://youtu.be/PnBnUUClclM

# The "Box" Pattern

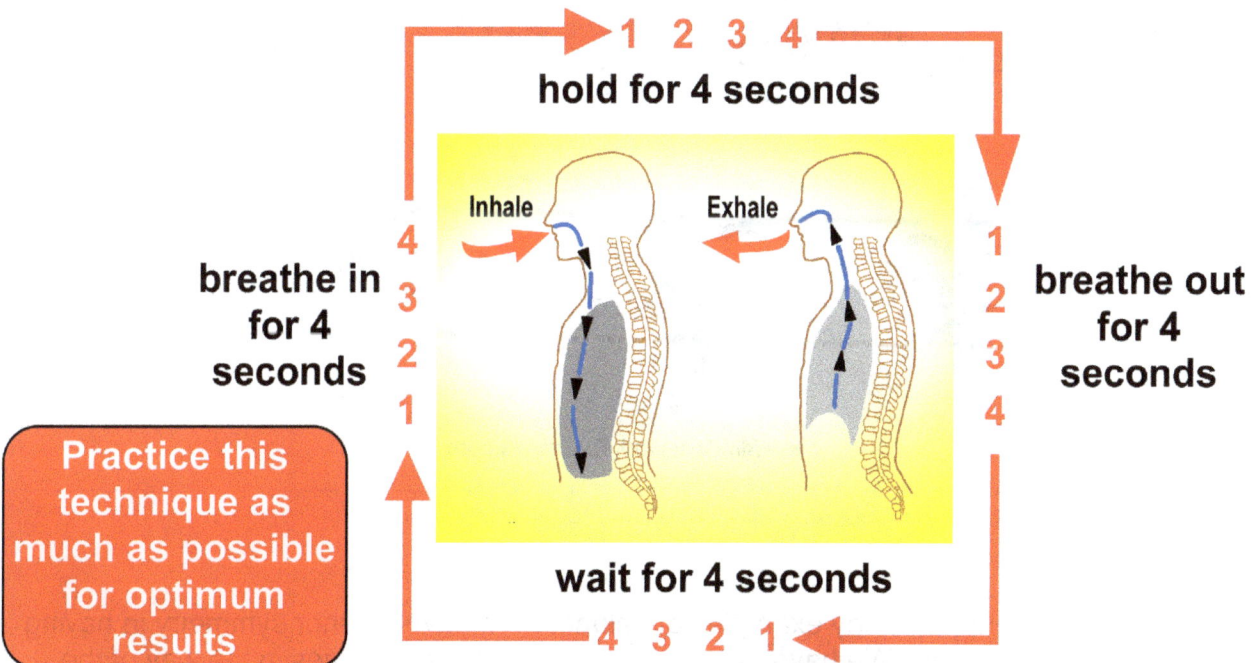

1 2 3 4
**hold for 4 seconds**

Inhale    Exhale

4
3
2
1
**breathe in for 4 seconds**

1
2
3
4
**breathe out for 4 seconds**

**wait for 4 seconds**
4 3 2 1

**Practice this technique as much as possible for optimum results**

## Can You Easily Stand on One Leg?

If you can easily stand and balance on one leg for more than a few seconds, chances are you can balance even better on two legs where you spend time standing, walking, running, etc. From my research, most people do not exercise or train themselves to improve or maintain balance *until an event presents itself* of where the individual loses their physical balance, stumbles, and/or falls and becomes injured. Then the search begins for them to find ways to improve their balance: physical therapy, medications or even refraining from activities that are now hazardous to the individual. The following is information I have gained from my own practicing and studying of martial arts and wellness methods spanning almost 40 years. Hopefully this will put readers on a path to achieving and maintaining better balance.

**A method to improve physical balance (vestibular) is to practice exercises that progressively challenge you to lose your sense of balance.**

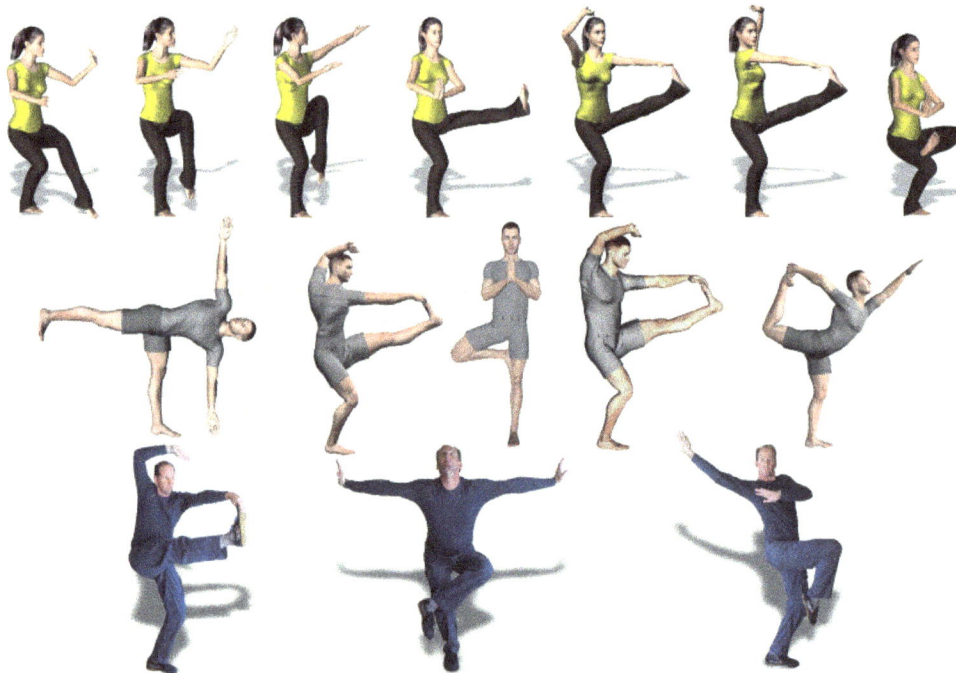

www.MindandBodyExercises.com

The human body contains many examples of balance. We have exterior symmetry in having 2 arms, 2 legs, 2 eyes, etc. We have interior symmetry within our bodies in the way of the muscular and skeletal systems being mostly equal from left to right side. The external body protects the internal organs, while the organs provide for the exterior. The mind governs the body while the body protects the mind. Vestibular balance is what most people think of as our spatial positioning and equilibrium in relation to standing, walking and general movement.

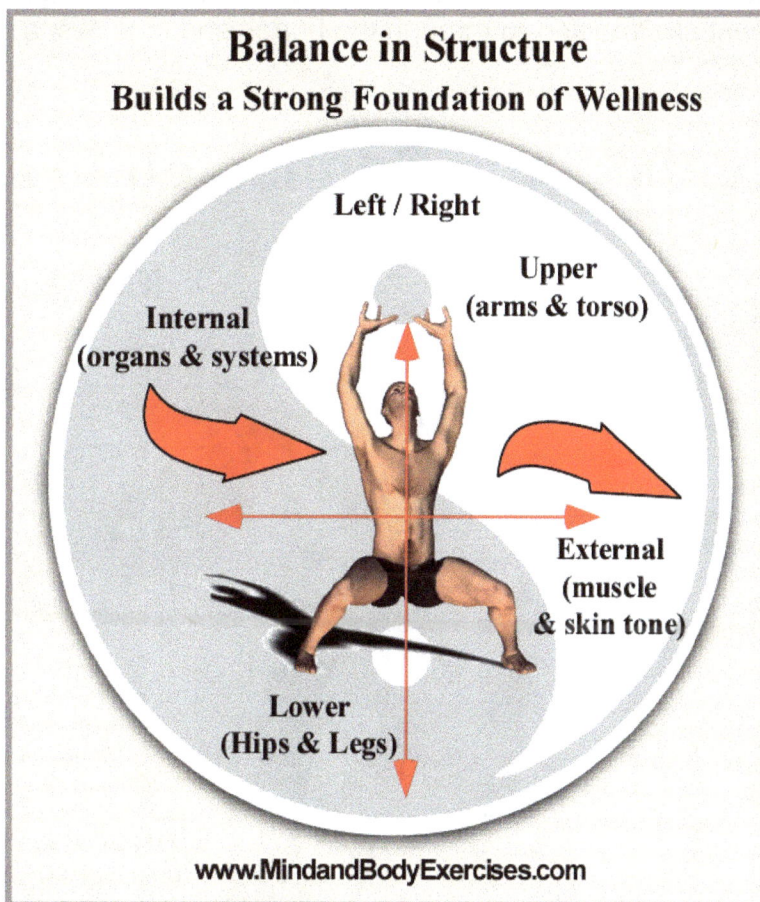

**Balance in Structure**
**Builds a Strong Foundation of Wellness**

Left / Right

Upper
(arms & torso)

Internal
(organs & systems)

External
(muscle
& skin tone)

Lower
(Hips & Legs)

www.MindandBodyExercises.com

Let's go into some basic anatomy and physiology relative to what allows the human body to not fall over with every movement we may execute.

**Body Components Connected to Balance**

**Brain** - the brain processes the signals from the eyes, inner ear and the sensory systems (skin, joints, muscles, nerves) of the human body.

**Eyes** - the eyes relate information to the brain such as spatial orientation and environmental conditions.

**Inner Ear** - the inner ear and the Vestibular system, regulates equilibrium while providing directional information to the brain to process.

**Sensory Receptor**s -nerves in the joints called proprioceptors, sense vibrations that flow through joints, muscles and skin sending the information to the brain to process.

10

## Osteoporosis (bone mass loss)

The last years of 2020 & 2021 were pretty rough years for most of the world population regarding health and wellness. While some people fared ok, many took many steps backward in being healthy and well. The exact measures many people have been taking to stay safe have actually contributed to them becoming less healthy. Staying inside dramatically affected positive social interactions, options to exercise and staying active, fresh air intake as well as less sunlight on the skin to help synthesize vitamin D. Vitamin D is a key component to maintain innate (natural immunity) and bone health. This issue alone will contribute to an increase in osteoporosis.

Osteoporosis, or low bone mass, is a disease that causes bones to become thin, brittle and weak, making bones more likely to break, most often from a minor fall. The most common bones that are affected are the spine, wrist or hip. Osteoporosis is often called a "silent disease." You can't feel or see your bones getting thinner. Many people do not even know that they have thin bones until a bone breaks. Most people with this issue don't die from osteoporosis, but rather from complications that follow from falling or breaking brittle bones while out and about.

Osteoporosis is a major public health issue with an estimated 44 million Americans, or for more than half of those 50 or older. In the United States, almost 1 out of 2 Caucasian or Asian women over 50 will experience a broken bone due to osteoporosis. 24 percent of hip fracture patients aged 50 and over die in the year following the fracture. Six months after a hip fracture, only 15 percent of patients can walk across a room unaided.

Things you can do to prevent loss of bone mass:
- A bone mineral density (BMD) test can diagnose osteoporosis.
- Eat a variety of healthy (nutrient-rich) foods every day.
- Get the calcium you need.
- Get the recommended amount of vitamin D.
- Get some sunlight on your body everyday (helps the body synthesize vitamin D)
- Don't smoke
- Limit alcohol.
- Take action to prevent falls
- Exercise regularly with appropriate methods for your personal situation, limits and expectations

Being physically active can help prevent bone loss leading to osteoporosis. Your bones get stronger and denser when you make them work. Walking, climbing stairs, and dancing are impact (or weight-bearing) exercises that strengthen your bones by moving your body against gravity when you are upright. Resistance exercises, such as lifting weights or using exercise bands, strengthen your bones as well as your muscles.

Tai Chi and qigong, like in the video linked below, are perfect examples of physical activity that improves posture and balance to help decrease your risk for falls and fractures. Tai chi can also strengthen the bones themselves by reacting to the tension that exercise puts on the muscles and consequently the bones.  If the bones are not engaged in everyday use, osteoporosis can find its way into the body. Exercise can be easy; try 10 minutes at a time, adding up the minutes to reach your goal.

https://youtu.be/Odi_GXzWTtI

_____

Osteoporosis and Osteopenia (bone porosity & bone loss)

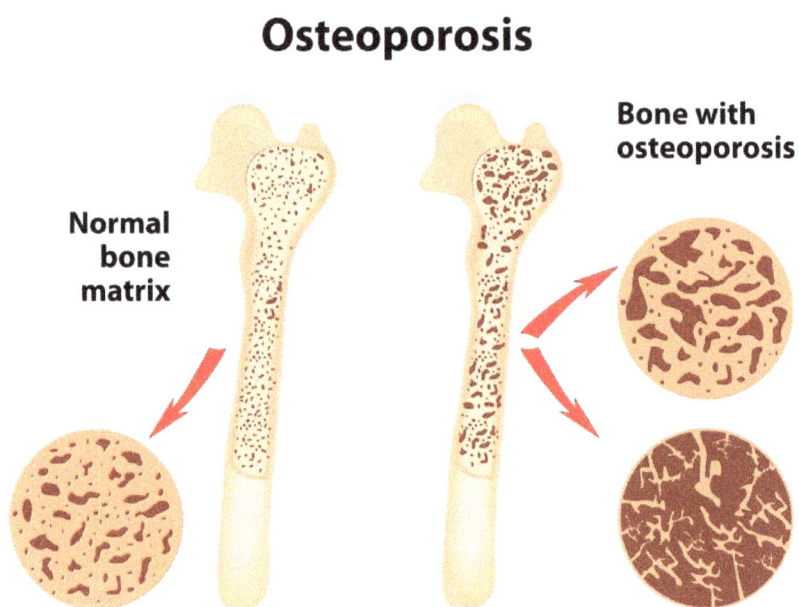

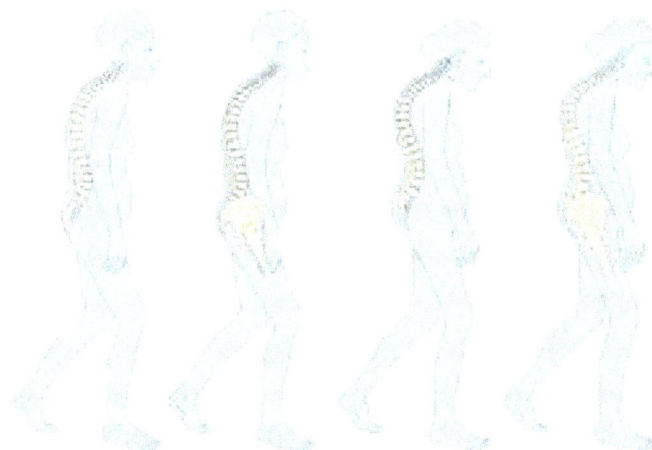

# Osteoporosis

Are you age 40 or older? If so, you might want to make sure you stay active as you continue to age. After 40 or so, the average woman losses 8% of their bone mass; men loss about 3% per decade. So, by 70 a woman can lose 25%; a man 18%. Bones can become more porous and weaker, usually starting to increase after age 45.

Wow, not good!

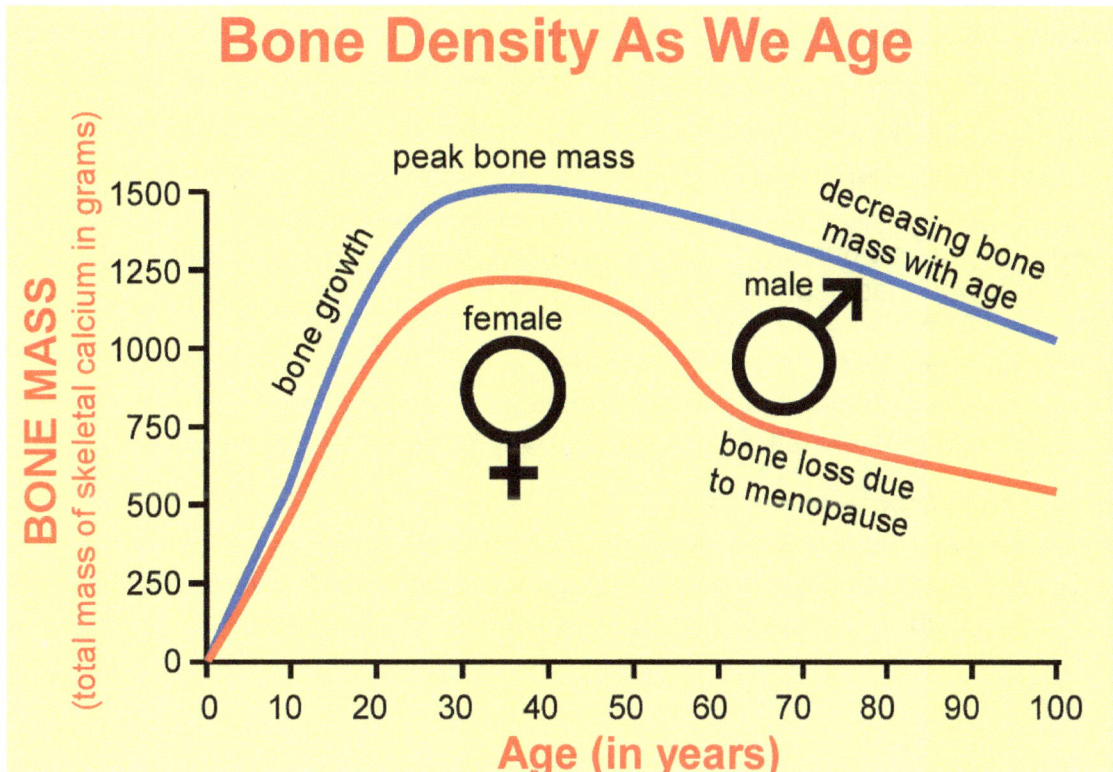

Consistent (and appropriate) exercise puts strain on the muscles, joints and bones, causing the bones cells to stay active and continue to remodel, often until the end of life. (Wolff's Law)Appropriate exercise as we all age depends upon the individual. However, Tai chi, yoga and qigong are all low-impact and can be practiced by most people regardless of age and health issues.

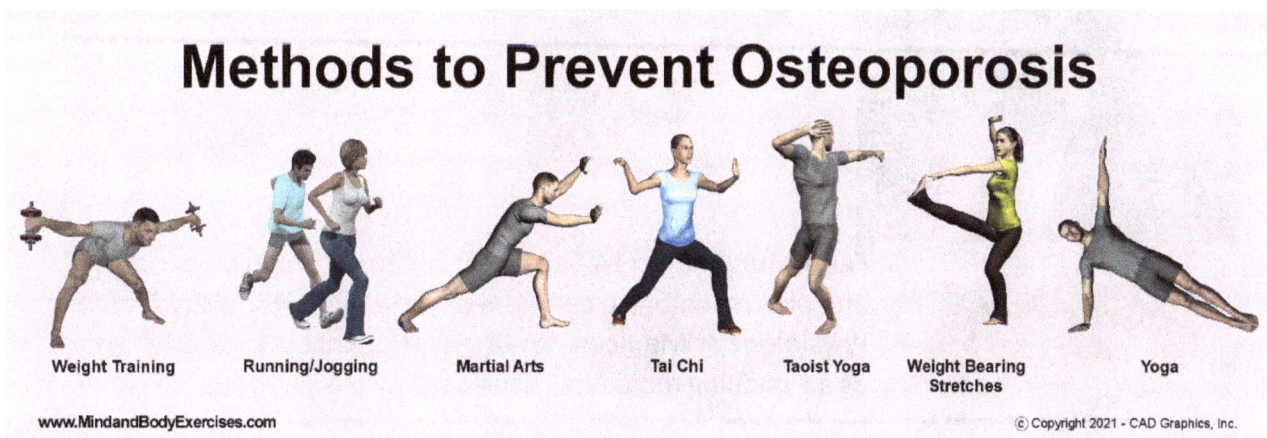

## Our Breath is the Link to the Mind-Body Connection

Our mental, physical and spiritual health – all comes down to the quality of our breath. Most people see their breath as an involuntary physiological process that they have little or no control over. While it is the first thing our bodies do when we are born and the last action before our physical body dies, there is a whole life of breathing in between. Every emotion affects the breath, just as managing breaths can affect the emotions, yin and yang in all things. Every respiration affects the body chemistry with hormones that are regulated by the "fight or flight" (sympathetic nervous system) and "rest and digest" (parasympathetic nervous system) mechanisms. Spending too much time in one zone or the other affects the balance of the nervous system, which affects organ functions, affecting the quality of life. Life is all about the breath and quality of it.

"Breath-work" is the new buzzword for mindful management of the breathing mechanism. Actually, breath-work has been practiced for thousands of years in methods from Yoga as Pranayama and its branches of qigong, as practiced through Traditional Chinese Medicine, tai chi and other martial arts.

Yogis and Buddhist practitioners of pranayama have long understood that our breath is an especially appropriate object of focus for meditation. The usage of the breath over other possible options has come about, presumably because respiration offers a readily available object to focus upon. Additionally, specific aspects of respiration can be observed as the breath adjusts in particular ways relative to emotions and attention (Wager & Cox, 2009). There are various types of Yogic breathing techniques of Pranayama, each offering differing benefits and goals. A few types would include long deep breathing, individual/alternating nostril breathing, and fast breathing.

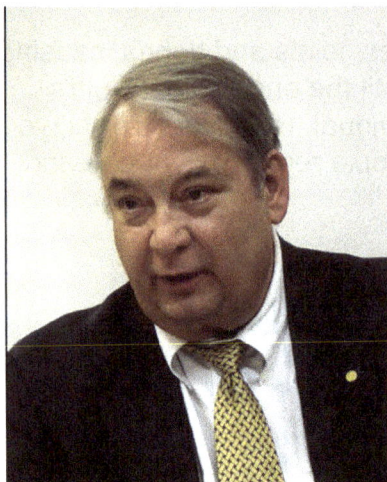

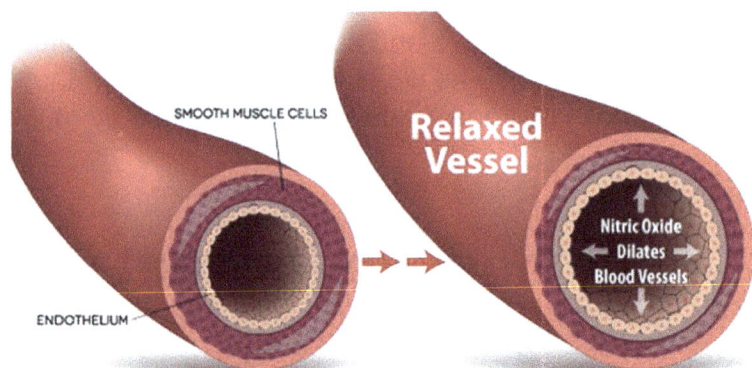

**Ferid Murat** (born 14 Sep 1936) Albanian origin physician and pharmacologist, co-winner of the 1998 Nobel Prize for Physiology or Medicine for discovering that nitric oxide, acts as a signalling molecule in the cardiovascular system.

September 14

# The Nobel Prize in Physiology or Medicine 1998

## The very first Signaling Molecule was discovered In 1998

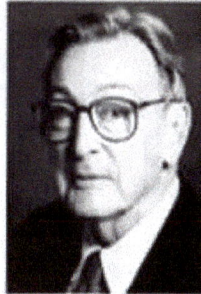

**Robert F. Furchgott**
Prize share: 1/3

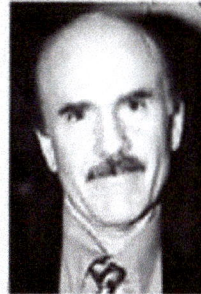

**Louis J. Ignarro**
Prize share: 1/3

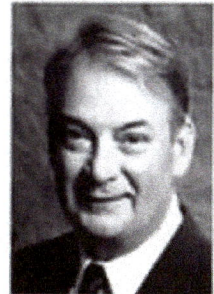

**Ferid Murad**
Prize share: 1/3

The Nobel Prize in Physiology or Medicine 1998 was awarded jointly to Robert F. Furchgott, Louis J. Ignarro and Ferid Murad *"for their discoveries concerning nitric oxide as a signalling molecule in the cardiovascular system".*

With managed and regulated breathing practices (such as pranayama, qigong and others), there is evidence that these practices create air oscillations which can increase nitric oxide (NO) through the rise in exchange of air between the nasal cavity and the paranasal sinuses. The paranasal sinuses can then produce larger amounts of nitric oxide which increases oxygen uptake. Nitric oxide aids in nonspecific host defense against infections stemming from bacteria, viruses, fungi, and parasites (Trivedi & Saboo, 2021). Nitric oxide was discovered in 1998 by Dr Robert F. Furchgott, Louis J. Ignarro and Ferid Murad for which they were awarded a Nobel prize. Nitric Oxide (NO) is a molecule that is produced in the nose naturally, as well as throughout the human body. NO has anti-inflammatory, antiviral, antibacterial effects. NO is a very strong vasodilator that causes blood vessels to dilate (widen) while also stimulating the certain hormones to be released, such as human growth hormone and insulin. Nitric oxide is also used as a pharmacological inhalant as well for various other ailments (India, 2020).

**Sympathetic Nervous System**
**"Fight or Flight"**

**Parasympathetic Nervous System**
**"Rest & Digest"**

Pupils Dilate

Inhibits Flow of Saliva

Accelerates Heartbeat

Dilates Bronchi

Inhibits Peristalsis & Secretion

Conversion of Glycogen to Glucose

Secretion of Adrenaline & Noradrenaline

Inhibits Bladder Contraction

Medulla Oblongata

$C_1$

$T_1$

$L_1$

$S_1$

Cardiac Plexus

Celiac Plexus

Mesentric Plexus

Chain of Sympathetic Ganglia

Ganglion

Vagus Nerve

Pupils Constrict

Stimulates Flow of Saliva

Slows Heartbeat

Constricts Bronchi

Stimulates Peristalsis & Secretion

Stimulates Release of Bile

Contracts the Bladder

Neurotransmitters secreted in SNS: (stress hormones)  Cortisol  Norepinephrine

Neurotransmitters secreted in PNS: ("happy" hormones)  Dopamine  Oxytocin  Seratonin  Endorphins

www.MindandBodyExercises.com

© Copyright 2021 - CAD Graphics, Inc

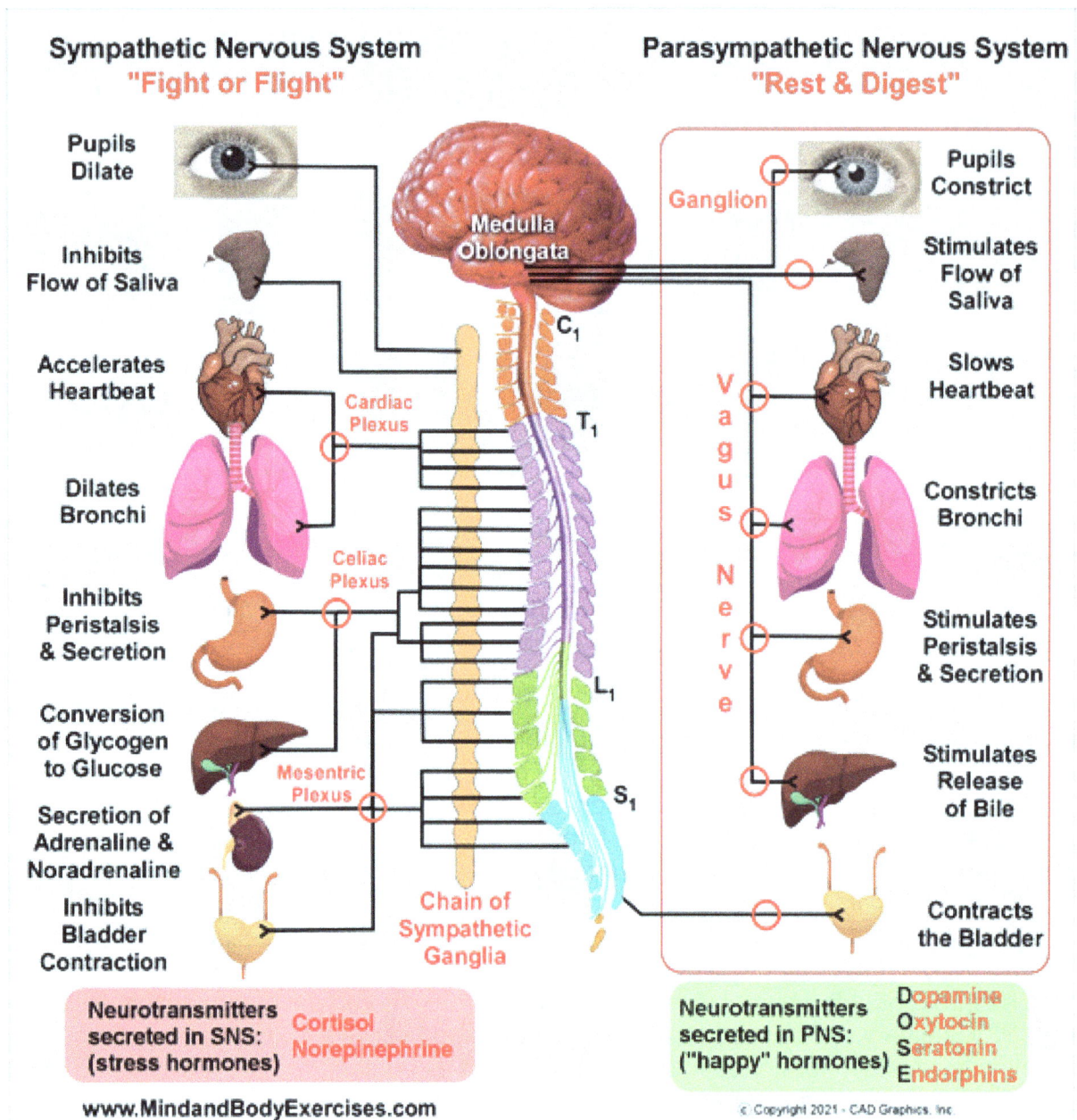

Our breath is the driving force of the spirit. People get caught up on the word "spirit" and often gravitate towards it being religious in its meaning. I understand (and teach) spirit as being one's self-awareness and further, the awareness that we are not our thoughts but rather the observer to our thoughts. Monitoring and observing our breath allow the individual into the window of their thoughts. Often people will say that they are mad, sad, happy or other emotional states. Really, they are none of these things but rather experiencing anger, sadness, happiness, etc. An example would be when we see something disturbing come about and we can take a few slow deep breaths and then consciously engage our thoughts to think, "*NO I'm not going to engage in negative thoughts.*" Maybe we change the environment or conversation thereby making it upbeat and positive. We can consciously change our thought patterns.

# Thoughts Affect Your Organs

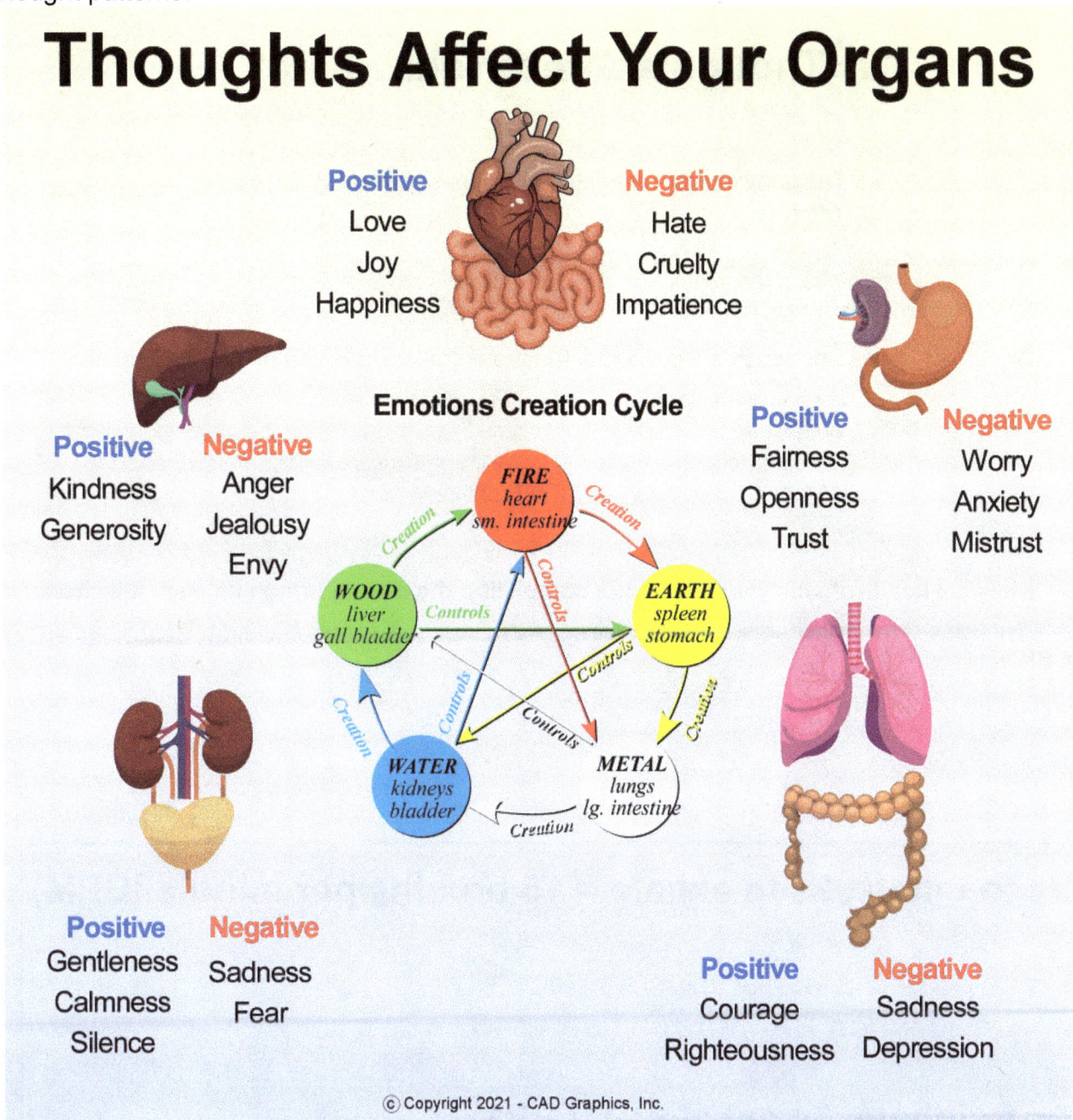

**Positive**
Love
Joy
Happiness

**Negative**
Hate
Cruelty
Impatience

**Positive**
Fairness
Openness
Trust

**Negative**
Worry
Anxiety
Mistrust

**Positive**
Kindness
Generosity

**Negative**
Anger
Jealousy
Envy

## Emotions Creation Cycle

*FIRE*
*heart*
*sm. intestine*

*WOOD*
*liver*
*gall bladder*

*EARTH*
*spleen*
*stomach*

*WATER*
*kidneys*
*bladder*

*METAL*
*lungs*
*lg. intestine*

*Creation*
*Controls*

**Positive**
Gentleness
Calmness
Silence

**Negative**
Sadness
Fear

**Positive**
Courage
Righteousness

**Negative**
Sadness
Depression

The breathwork can be addressed on the physiology level too, to get the conversation away from the religious or metaphysical aspects of being spiritual. In this narrative we can understand that the monitoring and regulating of the breath affects the thoughts which can affect our emotions, which affects the autonomic nervous system and thereby adjusts the blood chemistry and internal organs and their functions, which circles back to affecting our moods and thoughts once again. So really, spirit (or self-awareness) can come down to chemistry and how we can use it as a tool to reach our goals, whether physical, mental or spiritually based.

# Thoughts Affect Your Health

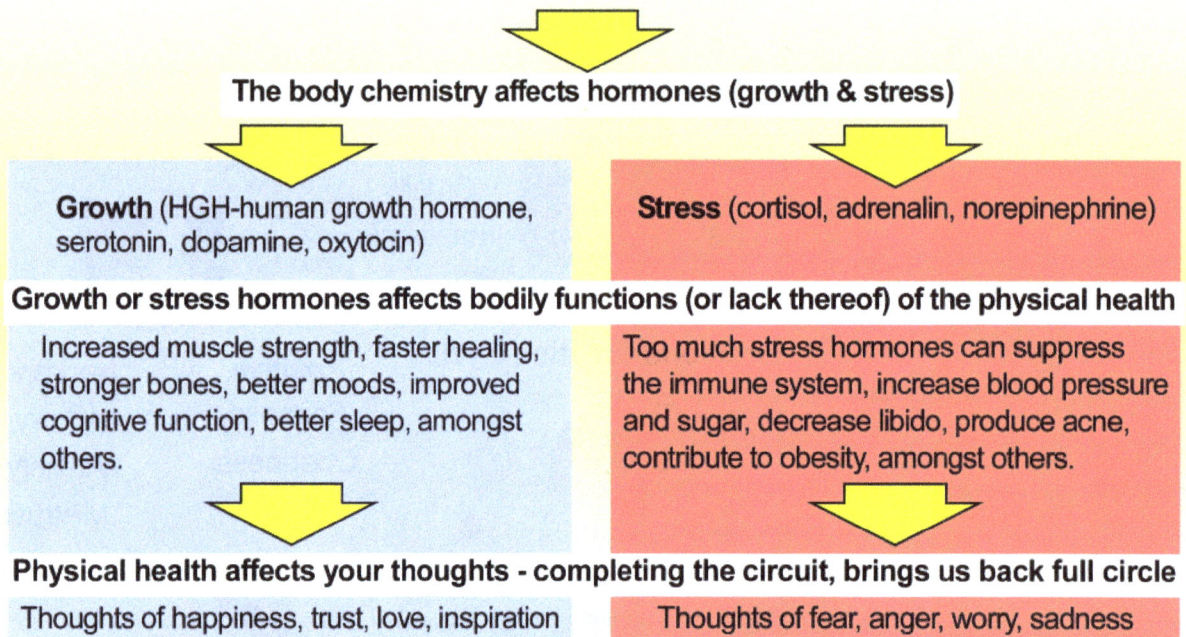

The body chemistry affects hormones (growth & stress)

**Growth** (HGH-human growth hormone, serotonin, dopamine, oxytocin)

**Stress** (cortisol, adrenalin, norepinephrine)

Growth or stress hormones affects bodily functions (or lack thereof) of the physical health

Increased muscle strength, faster healing, stronger bones, better moods, improved cognitive function, better sleep, amongst others.

Too much stress hormones can suppress the immune system, increase blood pressure and sugar, decrease libido, produce acne, contribute to obesity, amongst others.

Physical health affects your thoughts - completing the circuit, brings us back full circle

Thoughts of happiness, trust, love, inspiration

Thoughts of fear, anger, worry, sadness

**2s to inhale, 2s to exhale = 15 breaths per minute (BPM)**

**parasympathetic nervous system engages when BPM drops below 10**

**3s to inhale, 3s exhale = 10 BPM**

**4s to inhale, 4s exhale = 7.5 BPM**

Toned arms, a flat stomach, a well sculpted physique - are all very nice to have at the very least on the cosmetic level. However, lack of these are not the leading causes of death. Healthy internal organs and their various bodily functions are the foundation of wellness.

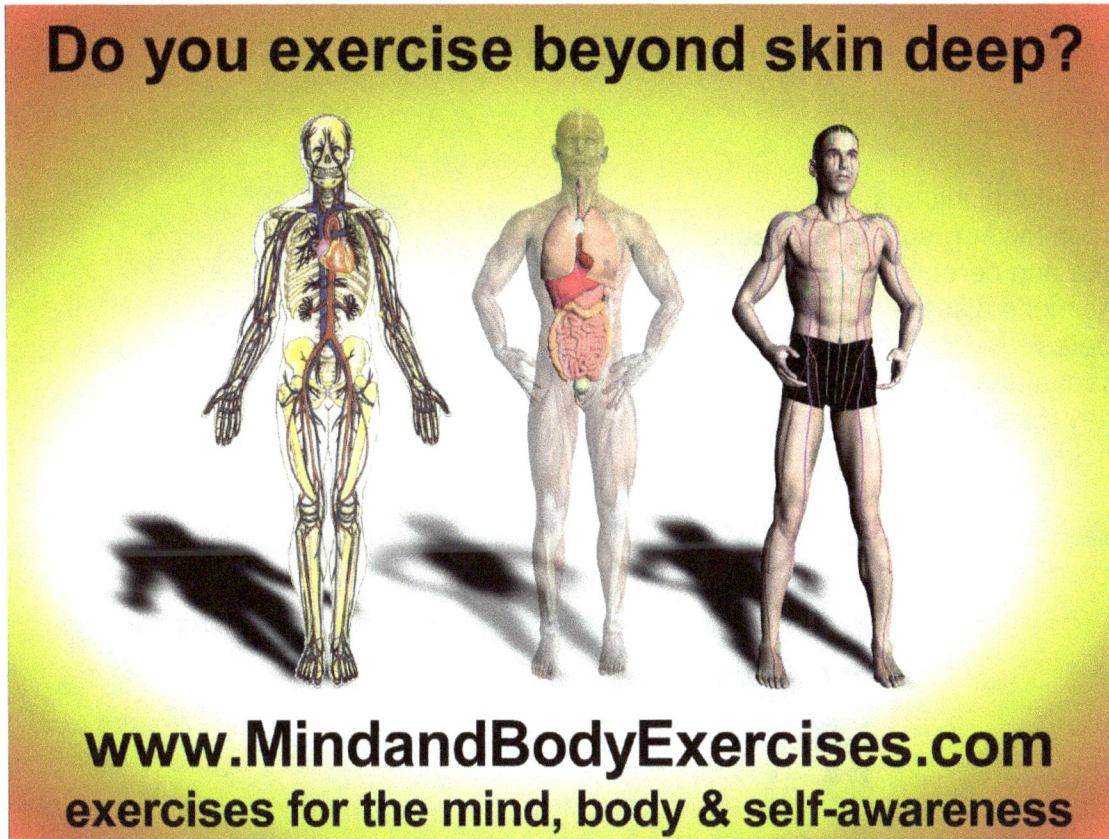

Do you exercise beyond skin deep?

www.MindandBodyExercises.com
exercises for the mind, body & self-awareness

There are major differences between fitness, health and wellness.

**Fitness** focuses on your physical health including nutrition, strength, conditioning, flexibility, and body composition with specific markers based on body size, gender, body type, training style, and training age. Fitness is a component of wellness, but wellness isn't a component of fitness.

**Health** is a state of being – physical, mental, and social well-being. Primary determinants of health include the social, economic, and physical environments, and individual characteristics and behaviors.

**Wellness (well-being)** includes fitness but it's broader. Wellness considers all of your choices and how they create your entire lifestyle. Wellness includes many facets and looks at the way they interact to create balance or imbalance. Think of wellness as a web, then plucking it one part creates reverberations across the rest.

Wellness is the state of living a healthy lifestyle. Wellness is considered a conscious, self-directed and evolving process of achieving full potential. Wellness is multidimensional and holistic, encompassing lifestyle, mental and spiritual well-being, and the environment. Wellness is finding a balance between all of these and enhancing a sense of happiness.

### The leading causes of death in the US for 2017-2018 (from the CDC):

1) Heart Disease
2) Cancer
3) Unintentional injuries
4) Chronic lower respiratory disease
5) Stroke and cerebrovascular diseases
6) Alzheimer's disease
7) Diabetes
8) Influenza and pneumonia
9) Kidney disease
10) Suicide

Figure 2. Age-adjusted death rates for all causes and the 10 leading causes of death in 2018: United States, 2017 and 2018

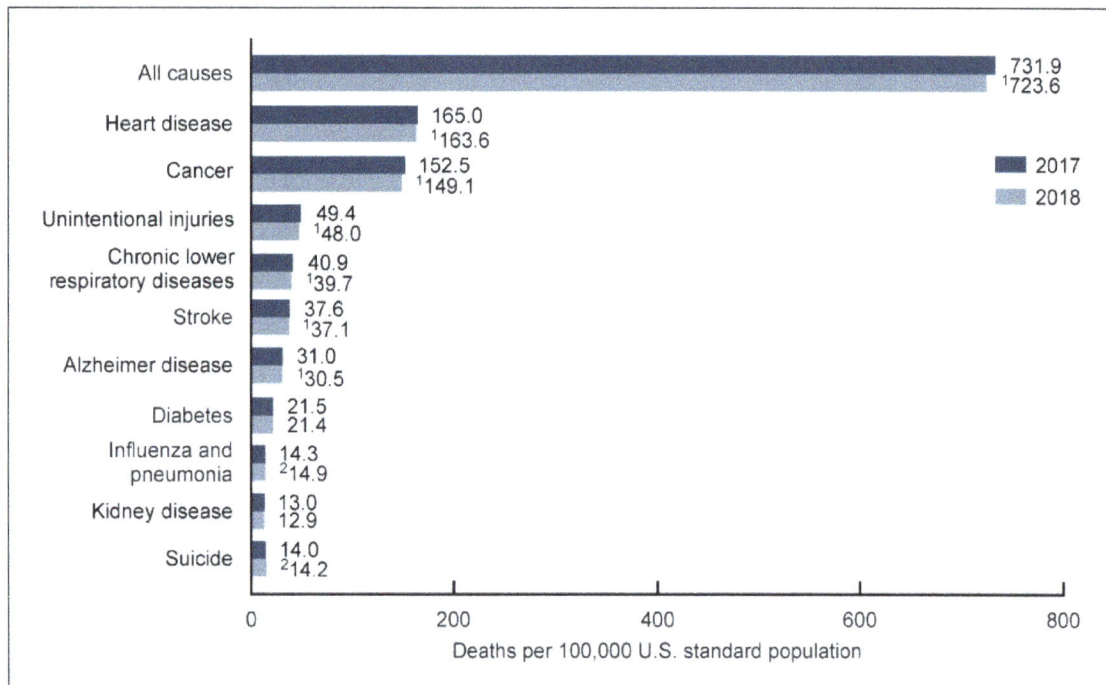

[1]Statistically significant decrease in age-adjusted death rate from 2017 to 2018 ($p < 0.05$).
[2]Statistically significant increase in age-adjusted death rate from 2017 to 2018 ($p < 0.05$).
NOTES: A total of 2,839,205 resident deaths were registered in the United States in 2018. The 10 leading causes of death accounted for 73.8% of all deaths in the United States in 2018. Causes of death are ranked according to number of deaths. Rankings for 2018 were the same as in 2017. Data table for Figure 2 includes the number of deaths for leading causes. Access data table for Figure 2 at: https://www.cdc.gov/nchs/data/databriefs/db355_tables-508.pdf#2.
SOURCE: NCHS, National Vital Statistics System, Mortality.

**The path to good or poor health doesn't happen overnight.**

# pH Balance & Effects

pH stands for "power of hydrogen."

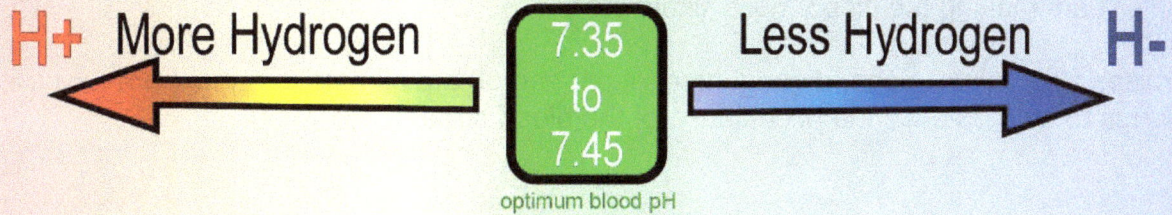

**H+**  More Hydrogen ←

7.35 to 7.45
optimum blood pH

Less Hydrogen →  **H-**

## More Acidic          Neutral          More Alkaline

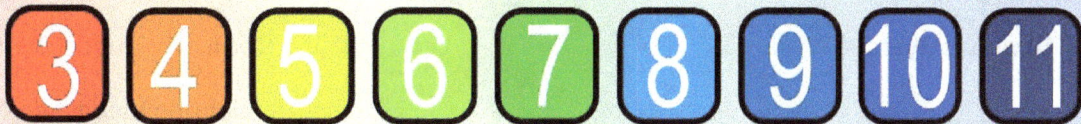

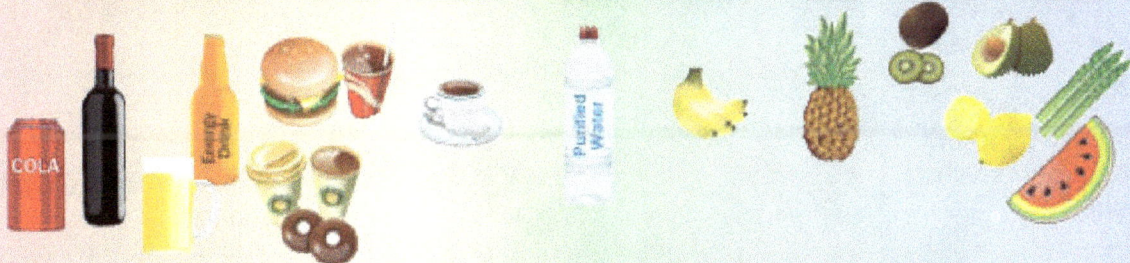

3  4  5  6  7  8  9  10  11

COLA · Energy Drink

Purified Water

## Acidosis
**Cause:**
acidic foods, soda, alcohol, cheeses, energy drinks, animal proteins, stress, aging, negative emotions, shallow breathing

## Wellness
**Enhanced by:**
water, alkaline foods, raw vegetables, fruits, positive emotions, deeper breathing

## Akalosis
**Cause:**
overabundance of bicarbonate in the blood, decreased blood levels of $CO_2$, or a loss of acid from the blood

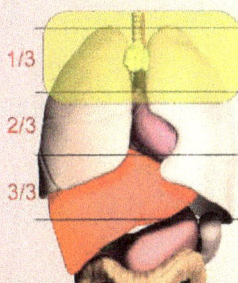

1/3
2/3
3/3

The respiratory system is also involved in balancing blood pH. More oxygen in the blood makes the pH less acidic and more alkaline.

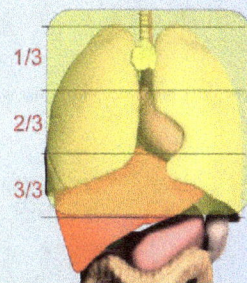

1/3
2/3
3/3

shallow breathing - top 1/3 of lung capacity (more $CO_2$ in blood)

deeper breathing - full lung capacity (more $O_2$ in the blood)

**www.MindandBodyExercises.com**

You are what you eat, think and how you move (or don't) move your body. If your diet is mostly acidic foods, your organs and all systems adjust. An acid-based diet is a cause of obesity, diabetes, heart disease, high blood pressure, and many more issues.

Shallow breathing, from stress and aging also allows for more carbon dioxide in the blood, which again is acidic to the blood and organs. Deeper breathing brings more oxygen into the blood stream making the blood more alkaline.

Exercises from tai chi, yoga, qigong, meditation, and others all help to bring more oxygen into the lungs to help balance the pH balance of the blood stream.

**SYMPTOMS OF ACIDOSIS**

**Central Nervous System**
Headache
Sleepiness
Confusion
Loss of consciousness
Coma

**Respiratory System**
Shortness of breath
Coughing

**Heart**
Arrhythmia
Increased heart rate

**Muscular System**
Seizures
Weakness

**Digestive System**
Nausea
Vomiting
Diarrhea

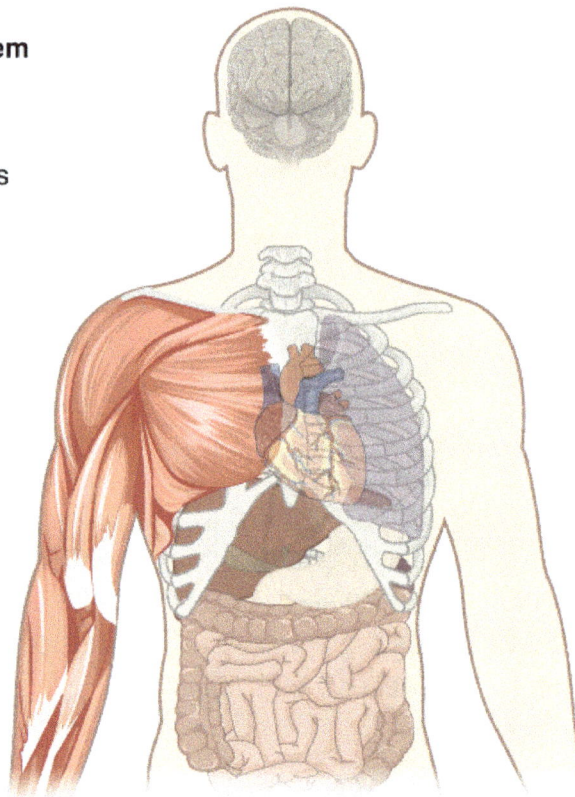

**SYMPTOMS OF ALKALOSIS**

**Central Nervous System**
Confusion
Light-headedness
Stupor
Coma

**Peripheral Nervous System**
Hand tremor
Numbness or tingling in
the face, hands, or feet

**Muscular System**
Twitching
Prolonged spasms

**Digestive System**
Nausea
Vomiting

*https://commons.wikimedia.org/wiki/File:2716_Symptoms_of_Acidosis_Alkalosis.jpg*

A root concept of healthcare for literally thousands of years, but apparently dismissed for the last 2 years:

**PHYSICAL ACTIVITY HELPS TO PREVENT DISEASE AND ILLNESS**
Become a researcher of health and wellness for your own benefit. Click on any of the following medical studies, to understand and then perhaps follow the science as to why physical activity & exercise are even more important today than maybe any other time before.
https://www.ncbi.nlm.nih.gov/pmc/articles/PMC7361852/

the british
psychological society
promoting excellence in psychology

Psychology and Psychotherapy: Theory, Research and Practice (2020)
© 2020 The Authors. Psychology and Psychotherapy: Theory, Research and Practice
published by John Wiley & Sons Ltd on behalf of British Psychological Society

www.wileyonlinelibrary.com

*Brief Report*

# Physical activity in a pandemic: A new treatment target for psychological therapy

Rowan Diamond[1,2,3]* and Felicity Waite[1,3]
[1]Department of Psychiatry, University of Oxford, UK
[2]Oxford Cognitive Therapy Centre, UK
[3]Oxford Health NHS Foundation Trust, UK

The COVID-19 pandemic and its management are placing significant new strains on people's well-being, particularly those with pre-existing mental health conditions. Physical activity has been shown to improve mental as well as physical health. Increasing activity levels should be prioritized as a treatment target, especially when the barriers to exercise are greater than ever. Promoting physical activity has not traditionally been the remit of psychologists. Yet psychological theory and therapeutic techniques can be readily applied to address physical inactivity. We present theoretical perspectives and therapy techniques relating to (1) beliefs about physical activity, (2) motivation to be physically active, and (3) the sense of reward achieved through being physically active. We outline strategies to initiate and maintain physical activity during the COVID-19 pandemic, thereby benefitting mental and physical health. COVID-19 is demanding rapid and substantial change across the whole health care system. Psychological therapists can respond creatively by addressing physical activity, a treatable clinical target which delivers both mental and physical health benefits.

https://medicine.umich.edu/dept/psychiatry/michigan-psychiatry-resources-covid-19/your-lifestyle/importance-physical-activity-exercise-during-covid-19-pandemic

**MICHIGAN MEDICINE**
UNIVERSITY OF MICHIGAN

**DEPARTMENT OF PSYCHIATRY**

Site search

CONTACT US

SUPPORT US

Home » Michigan Psychiatry Resources for COVID-19 » For Your Lifestyle » Exercise

◄ For Your Lifestyle

Exercise

Grief and Loss

Nutrition

Sleep

MICHIGAN RESEARCH EXPERTS

**Our Faculty on Michigan Research Experts**

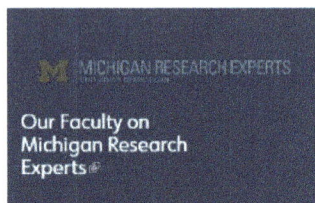

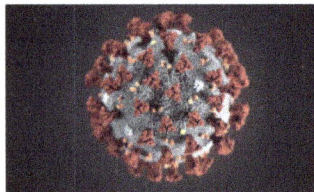

COVID-19 Mental Health Resources

# Importance of Physical Activity and Exercise during the COVID-19 Pandemic

## 3 Key Points

- Physical activity and exercise can be effective treatment strategies for symptoms of both depression and anxiety.
- Each day is a new opportunity to engage in physical activity and exercise that can bring short and long-term benefits for mood, sleep, and physical health.
- Consistency and sustained motivation may be enhanced by peer support, family support, or electronic platforms offering exercise programs.

British Journal of
**Sports Medicine**

Latest content    Current issue    Archive    Browse by collection    For authors

Home    Archive    Volume 55, Issue 19

Article Text

Article info

Citation Tools

Share

Rapid Responses

Article metrics

Alerts

PDF

PDF + Supplementary Material

Original research

## Physical inactivity is associated with a higher risk for severe COVID-19 outcomes: a study in 48 440 adult patients   FREE

Robert Sallis [1], Deborah Rohm Young [2], Sara Y Tartof [2], James F Sallis [3], Jeevan Sall [1], Qiaowu Li [2], Gary N Smith [4], Deborah A Cohen [2]

Correspondence to Dr Robert Sallis, Department of Family and Sports Medicine, Kaiser Permanente Medical Center, Fontana, CA 92335, USA; Robert.F.Sallis@kp.org

### Abstract

**Objectives** To compare hospitalisation rates, intensive care unit (ICU) admissions and mortality for patients with COVID-19 who were consistently inactive, doing some activity or consistently meeting physical activity guidelines.

**Methods** We identified 48 440 adult patients with a COVID-19 diagnosis from 1 January 2020 to 21 October 2020, with at least three exercise vital sign measurements from 19 March 2018 to 18 March 2020. We linked each patient's self-reported physical activity category (consistently inactive=0–10 min/week, some activity=11–149 min/week, consistently meeting guidelines=150+ min/week) to the risk of hospitalisation, ICU admission and death after COVID-19 diagnosis. We conducted multivariable logistic regression controlling for demographics and known risk factors to assess whether inactivity was associated with COVID-19 outcomes

**Results** Patients with COVID-19 who were consistently inactive had a greater risk of hospitalisation (OR 2.26, 95% CI 1.81 to 2.83),

*https://bjsm.bmj.com/content/55/19/1099*

A bimonthly publication part of the Brazilian Society of Cardiology portfolio of journals connected with ABC Cardiol publishing national and international scientific production in the field of cardiovascular sciences.

ISSN 2359-4802    eISSN 2359-5647

## ARTICLES

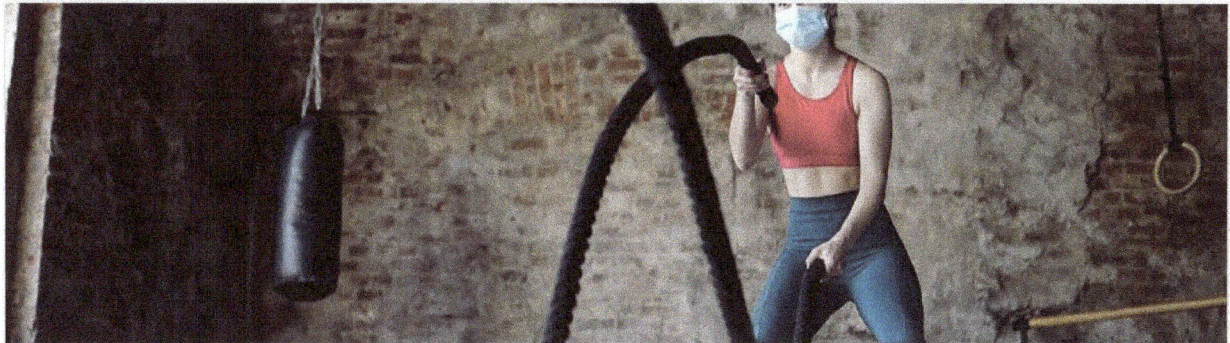

**LETTER TO THE EDITOR**

International Journal of Cardiovascular Sciences. 16/Apr/2021;34(3):324-5.

## The Big Mistake of not Considering Physical Activity an Essential Element of Care During the Covid-19 Pandemic

*Francisco José Gondim Pitanga* 🆔 , *Carmem Cristina Beck* 🆔 , *Cristiano Penas Seara Pitanga* 🆔

**DOI:** 10.36660/ijcs.20200274

Dear Editor,

In response to the letter to the editor entitled "Declaring physical activity as 'essential' during the Covid-19 pandemic may not be a good measure" that presented contributions to our point of view entitled "Should physical activity be considered essential activity during the Covid-19 pandemic?" we thank you for the suggestions and we present a reply letter with our arguments:

[...]

Poor circulation or Peripheral Arterial Disease (PAD) is the restriction of blood flow to the arteries of the arms and legs. When arteries become narrowed by the accumulation of cholesterol and other materials on the walls of the arteries also known as plaque, the oxygen-rich blood flowing through the arteries cannot reach the fingers and toes.

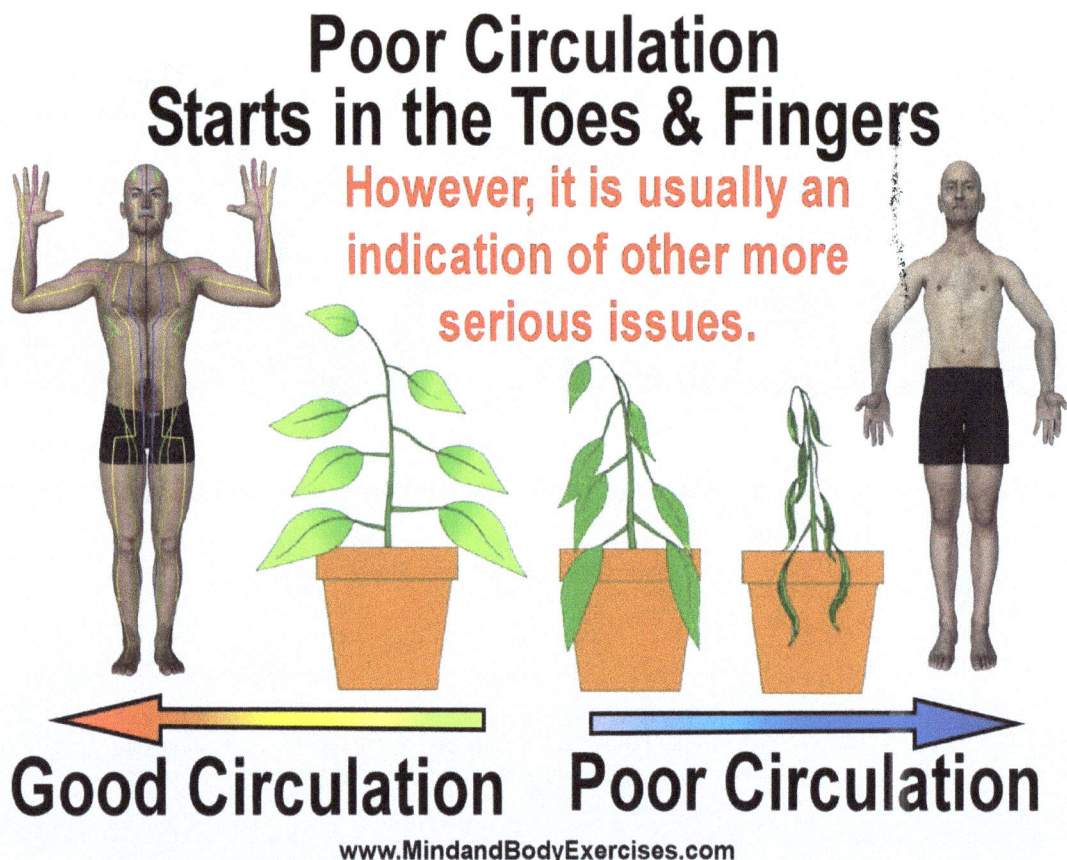

# Poor Circulation
## Starts in the Toes & Fingers

### However, it is usually an indication of other more serious issues.

## Good Circulation    Poor Circulation

www.MindandBodyExercises.com

As trees and plants age or lack water and nutrients, it becomes more difficult for the water to travel to the parts farthest from the roots, being the leaves and branches. This is why we see the leaves on trees and plants whither before they die. Just like a tree, our bodies have difficulty getting the blood to circulate to the farthest parts from the heart, being the fingers and toes. This concept leads to the thought that we need to pay extra attention towards the fingers and toes to ensure good blood circulation throughout the whole body.

Often people look for medicine to achieve this, when in reality a balanced diet and proper exercise can be the solution. Most people that do exercise usually don't focus specifically on exercising the toes and fingers and consequently still develop arthritis, rheumatism and other issues within the hands and feet. Tai Chi, qigong and yoga are methods that engage all parts of the body literally, from head to toe and not just the main muscle groups.

## Posture and Symmetry Affect the Body and Mind

Which side do you favor?
Do you have a stronger side?
A weaker side you avoid?
A faster side you use for activities?

Some of the above have to do with your posture and natural symmetry of your body.

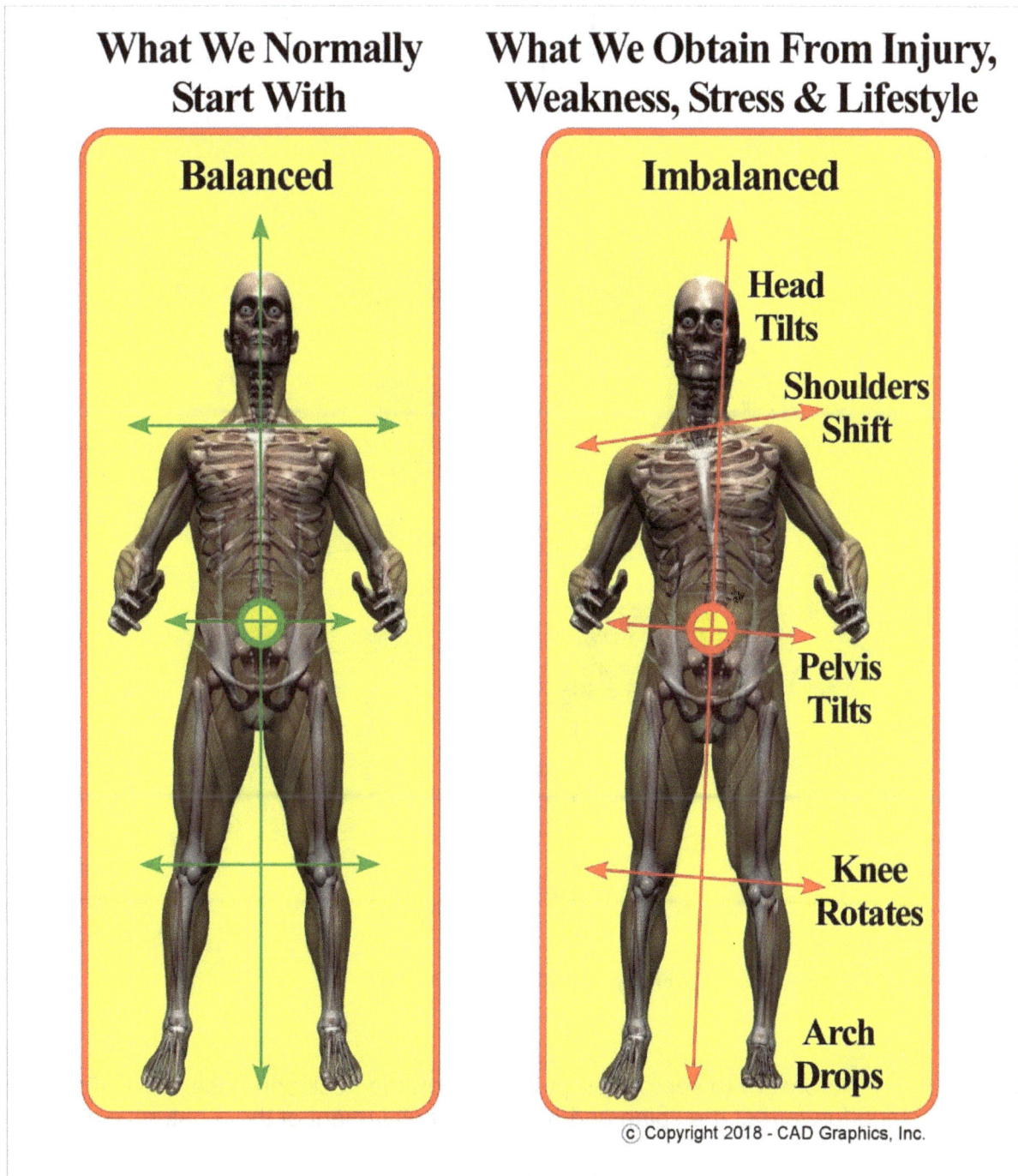

**What We Normally Start With** — Balanced

**What We Obtain From Injury, Weakness, Stress & Lifestyle** — Imbalanced: Head Tilts, Shoulders Shift, Pelvis Tilts, Knee Rotates, Arch Drops

© Copyright 2018 - CAD Graphics, Inc.

Most people in the United States will experience back pain at some time in their lives. Some find relief through options like rest, medications, exercise, stretching, chiropractic, acupuncture, physical therapy and sometimes surgery. Most pain goes away within a few days or weeks only to return at a later date. In many cases, the root cause of back pain is tight hamstring muscles. Excessive sitting or standing can tighten these muscles, as well as lack of proper stretching on a regular basis. Other root causes of back pain are many ranging from poor posture, heavy lifting, sports injuries, career, lack of exercise, congenital and others. **Unless the root cause is found and addressed, most treatments only offer temporary relief.**

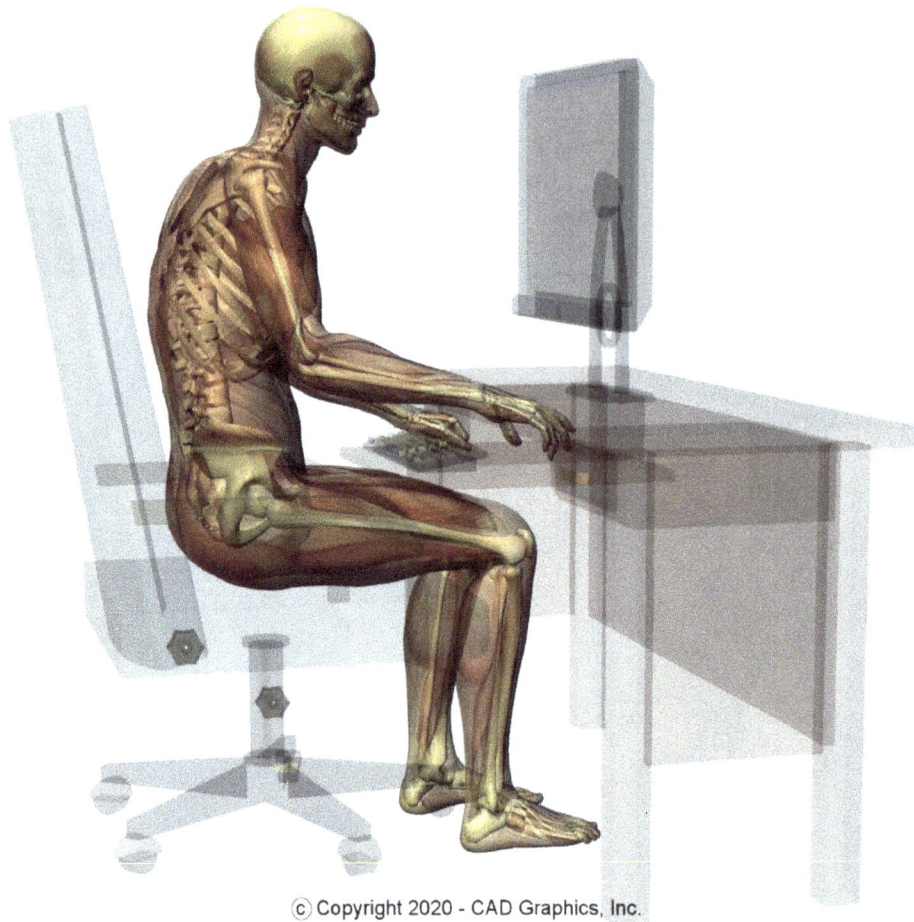

Straining the neck forward to see closer, puts strain on the neck and upper back. This leads to hunching forward of the spine and a gradual realignment of the 3 natural curves.

Poor posture, combined with long hours sitting stagnant in a chair cause muscles within the legs to shorten and tighten over time. These muscles, specifically the hamstrings, cause the pelvis to tilt the tailbone forward.

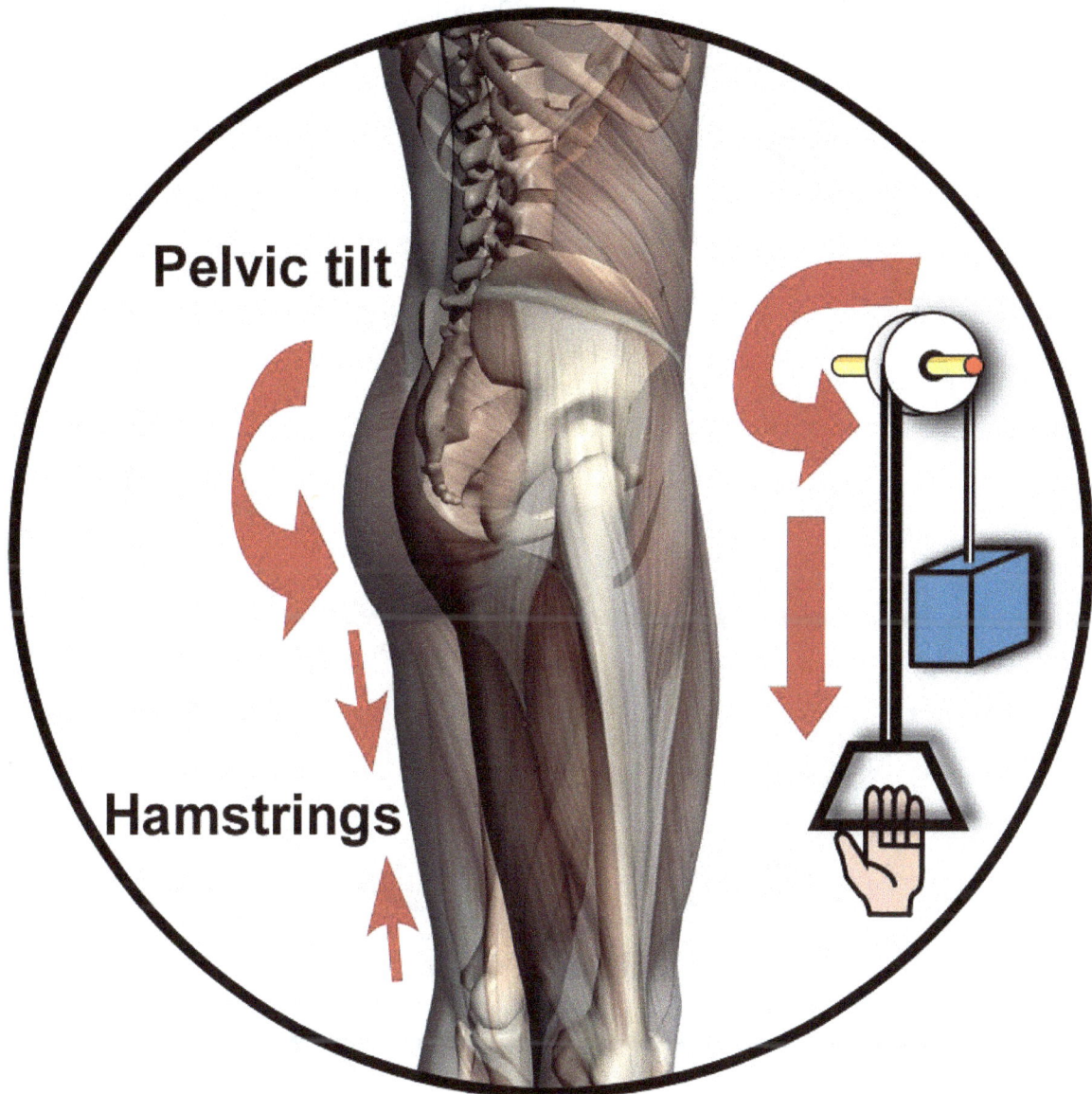

**Pelvic tilt**

**Hamstrings**

© Copyright 2020 - CAD Graphics, Inc.

Just like a pulley, the hips rotate towards the tight muscle groups. Tight hamstrings cause the pelvis to tilt the tailbone forward which put increased tension on lower back muscles.

Pelvic tilt also puts strain on the lower back muscles such as the quadratus lumborum. Spasm can occur as the muscles tighten even more to protect the spine from excessive movement. The piriformis muscle attaches the head of the femur to the base of the pelvis. The piriformis can become irritated or tense causing pain to the nearby sciatic nerve. Sciatica can cause pain and numbness down the back of the legs to the heels and toes.

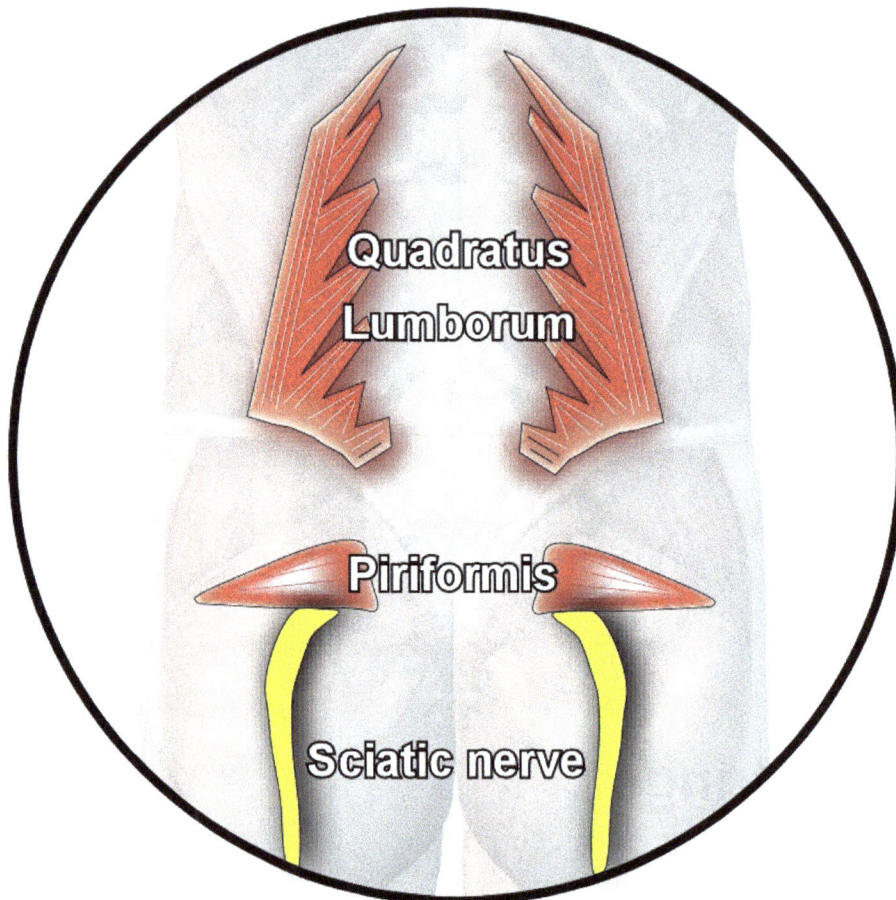

© Copyright 2020 - CAD Graphics, Inc.

The below set of exercises develop strength and flexibility which can improve posture. Good health of the lower back starts with good posture. Strength in the back, hips and abdomen provide a strong cage that houses the internal organs. Flexibility in these areas helps to maintain good blood circulation to the organs and lower body. Lengthening of the spine while exercising reduces stress and tension on the nervous system. Relax the body into the positions in spite of any tension in the muscles. Deep and relaxed breathing is essential while performing these exercises.

Try to match your body position similar to those as shown below. Don't be discouraged by not being able to achieve these stretches but rather do what your body is capable of. Stretches can be performed on the floor, on a mattress or even in a swimming pool or hot tub. Try for a few seconds in each position for a total of a few minutes. As your flexibility increases in the hamstrings, less tension will be placed on the lower back muscles. Try to do some of the exercises every day for at least a few days in a row. As the pain is relieved, try to add more time for each exercise working up to a total of a half-hour or full hour. As less pain is present, try to maintain a regular schedule of performing these exercises to keep the problem from recurring. All stretches should be performed on both sides.

## Seated toe touch

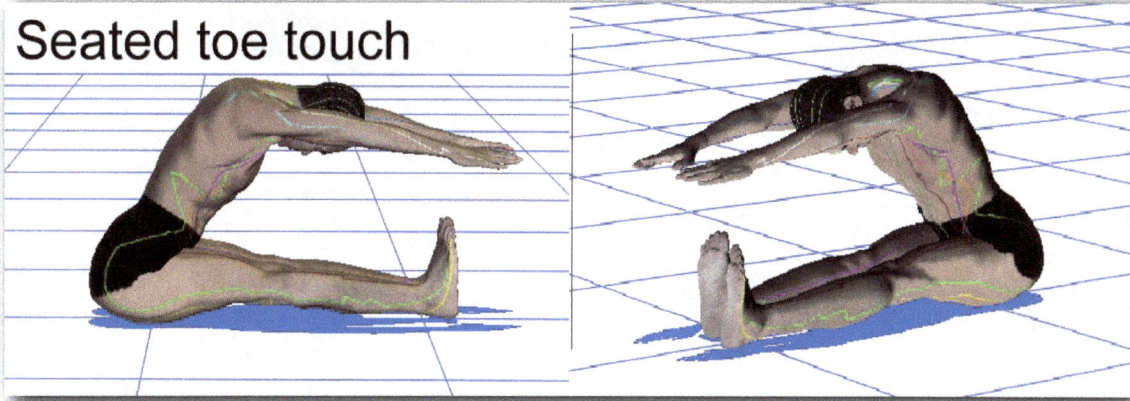

Sit on the buttocks as leaning the upper body forward. Focus more on the torso coming forward than the hands reaching the feet.

## Piriformis stretch

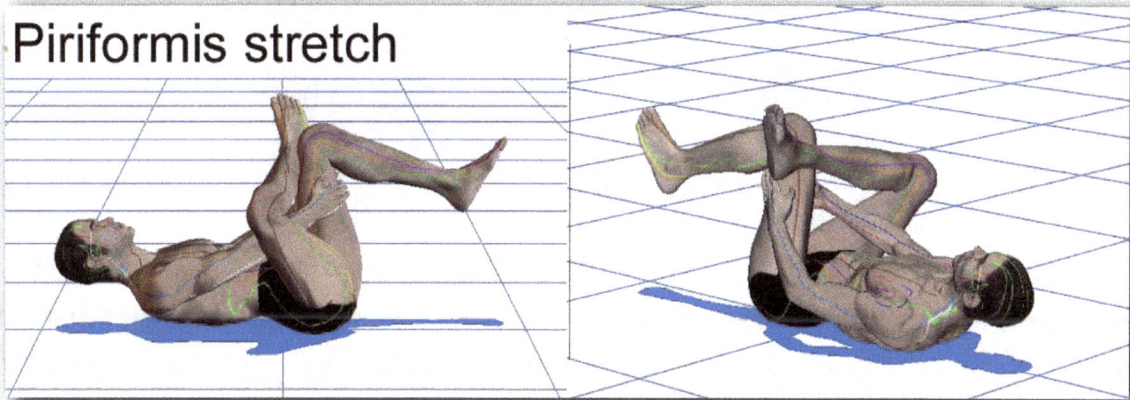

Lay flat on the back as bending both knees. Try to cross the right foot over the left knee. Pull the left leg towards your face as the right hip stretches

# Knee to opposite hand

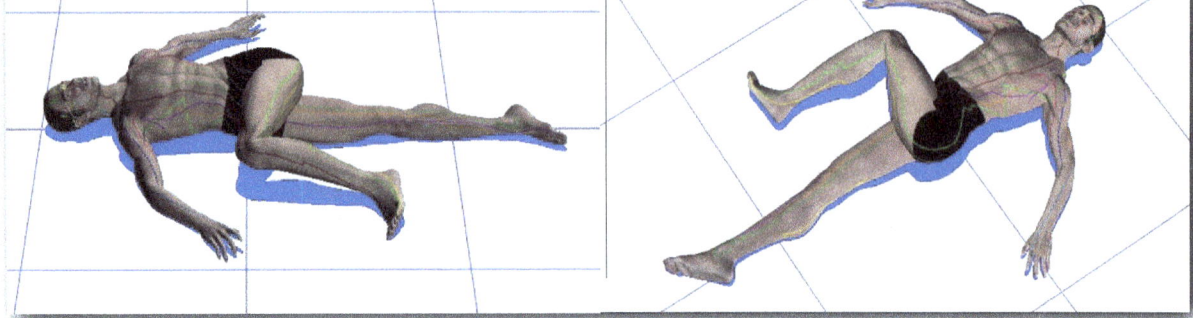

Lay flat on your back, bring a bent knee across the other straight leg. Relax the neck and arms as you feel the lower back stretch to the side.

# Standing toe touch

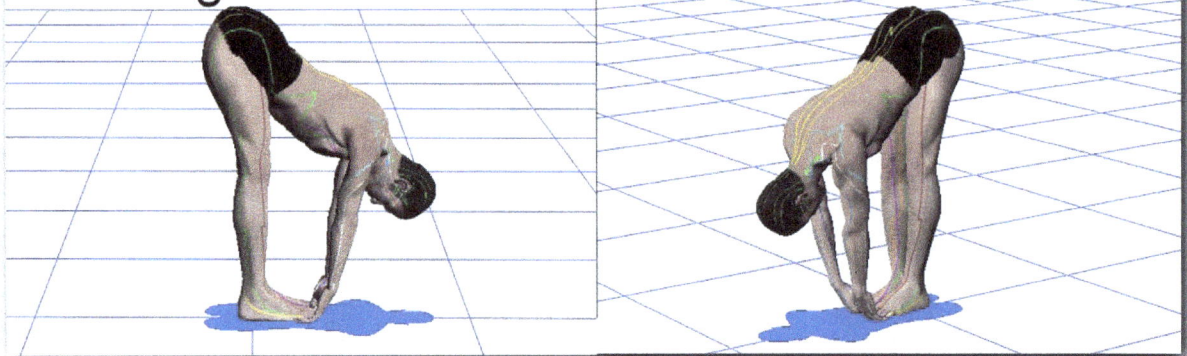

Feet together while bending forward at the waist. Reach as far downward as comfortable.

# Torso twist

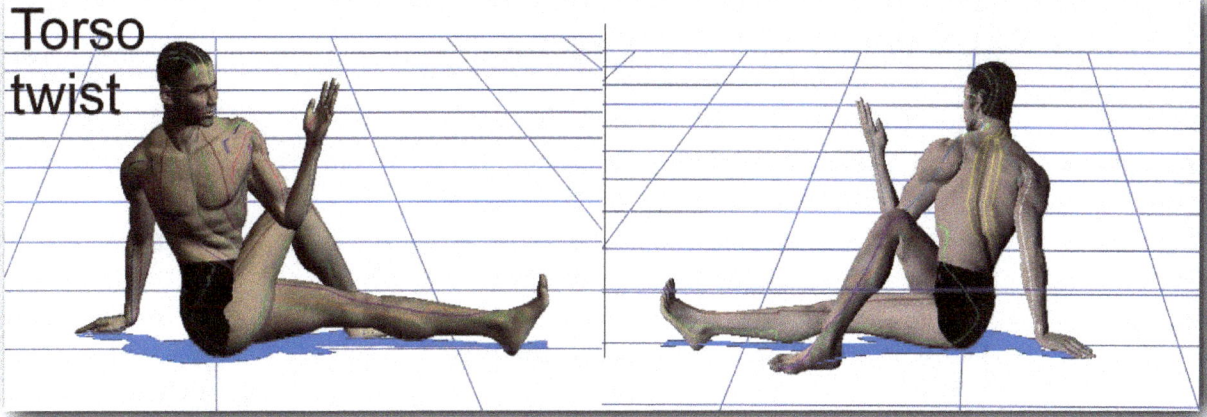

Sit on the buttocks with one leg straight and one leg bent and crossed over the other. Turn the upper body opposite while relaxing the back.

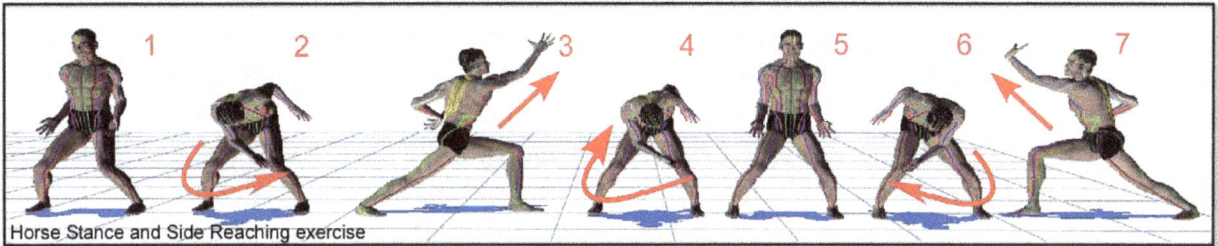

Horse Stance and Side Reaching exercise

Feet slightly wider than shoulder width, knees bent, hands open positioned next to the hips. Back straight, lower back arched inward as hips sinks down. Left Bo-stance as opposite arm extends out and away from back heel. Left hand, arm & shoulder twist with the torso towards the left. Sink hips. Alternate on both sides.

## Why do You Exercise?

Do you exercise for fitness, health, appearance, stress relief?

Another perspective might be to think about YOUR healthcare program being geared towards particular goals such as:

**Restoration** - regaining a prior level of healthy fitness

**Longevity** - utilizing exercises that align with one's age and current abilities without causing more harm than good.

**Cultivation** - practicing methods to sustain good health and conserve energy to be utilized in our latter years of life.

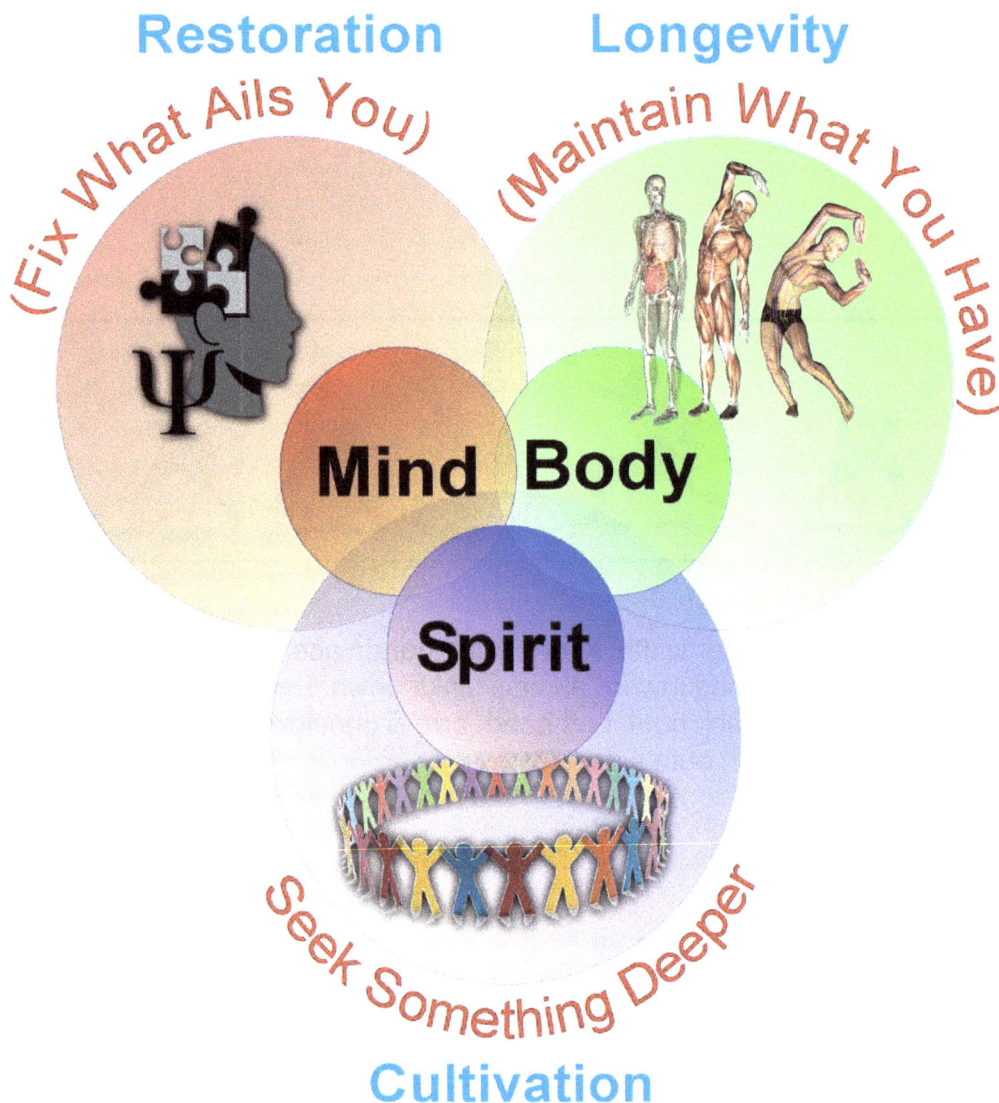

This is very similar to my recent post on knee pain. Back, knee, shoulder, neck - it really is the same basic issue. What is your plan?

# Sciatica - Pain in the Butt!

**Symptoms of Sciatica:**
- pain in lower back, hips, legs and/or feet
- burning, tingling, numbness, weakness

**Causes of Sciatica:**
- disc herniation        - obesity
- bone spurs            - injury
- postural imbalances
- tight muscular structure

**Treatments:**
- rest                  - pain meds
- chiropractic          - massage
- exercise              - therapy
- surgery               - acupuncture

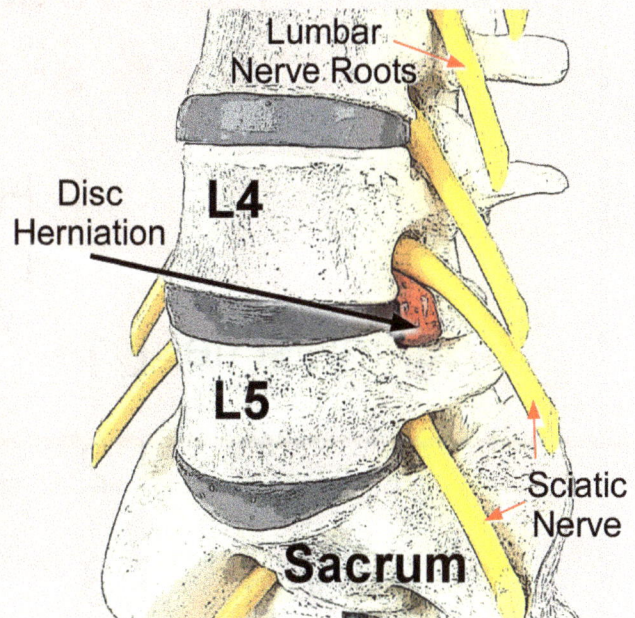

Lumbar Nerve Roots

Disc Herniation

L4

L5

Sciatic Nerve

Sacrum

**www.MindandBodyExercises.com**

Become educated should be number 1, no?

- Give it a rest? Sit, stand or lie down?
- Ice or heat? When is one more beneficial?
- Keep active? When do you decide to get moving again?
- Go to your doctor? Chiropractor, physical therapist? Alternative exercise coach?
- Get an x-ray? MRI?
- Medicate? Anti-inflammatories (NSAIDs), opioids?
- Surgery? Microdiscectomy, spinal fusion, epidural?

# Compressed Spine
# Can Affect Other Areas

The health of the spine affects the nervous, muscular, circulatory & skeletal systems

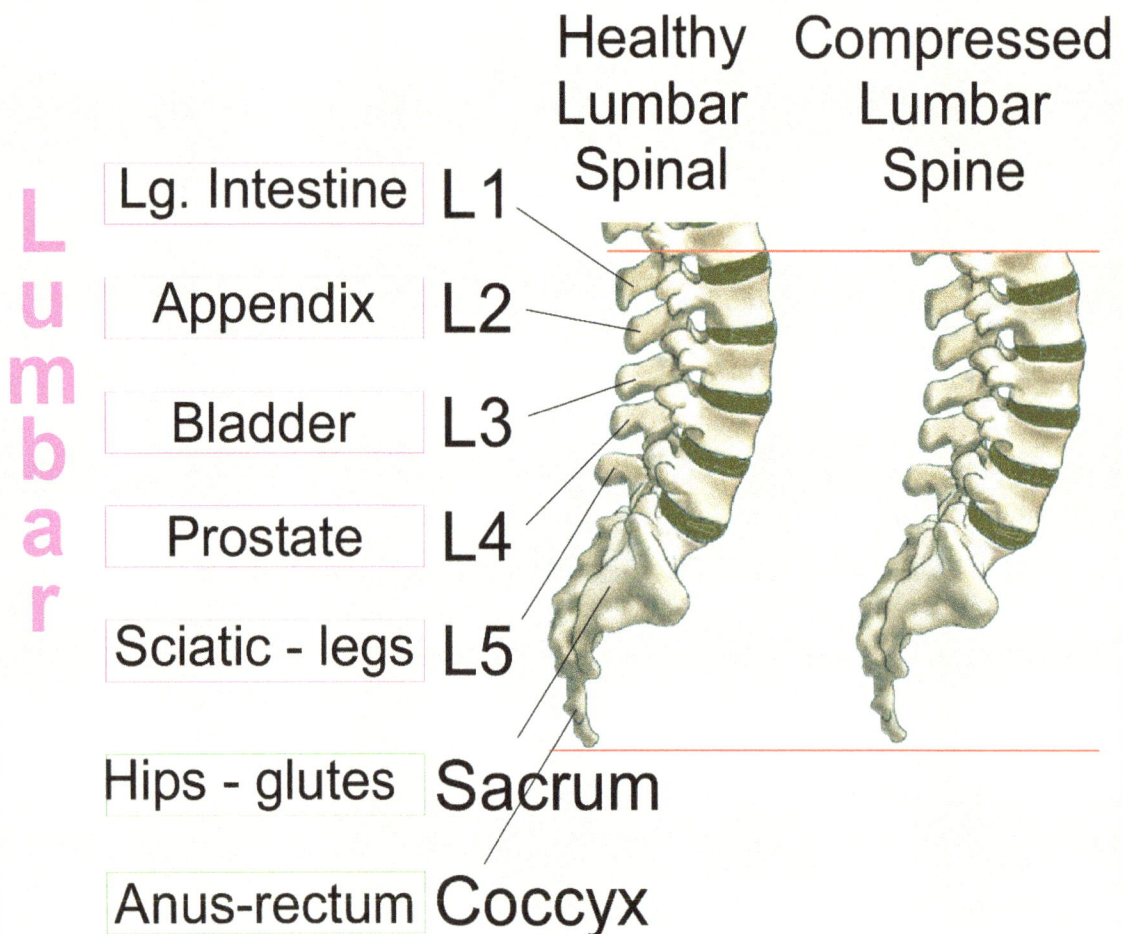

Healthy Lumbar Spinal | Compressed Lumbar Spine

**L**
**u**
**m**
**b**
**a**
**r**

| Lg. Intestine | L1 |
| Appendix | L2 |
| Bladder | L3 |
| Prostate | L4 |
| Sciatic - legs | L5 |
| Hips - glutes | Sacrum |
| Anus-rectum | Coccyx |

## www.MindandBodyExercises.com

105

Depending upon your issues, maybe yes to all of the above. Without knowing how serious your injury is, it can be difficult to plot a course to relieve the pain and gain back confidence in your activities. You need to do the homework and research to become educated as to what injuries are typical and what the options are to move forward.

# Sciatica - One Part Affects Other Parts!

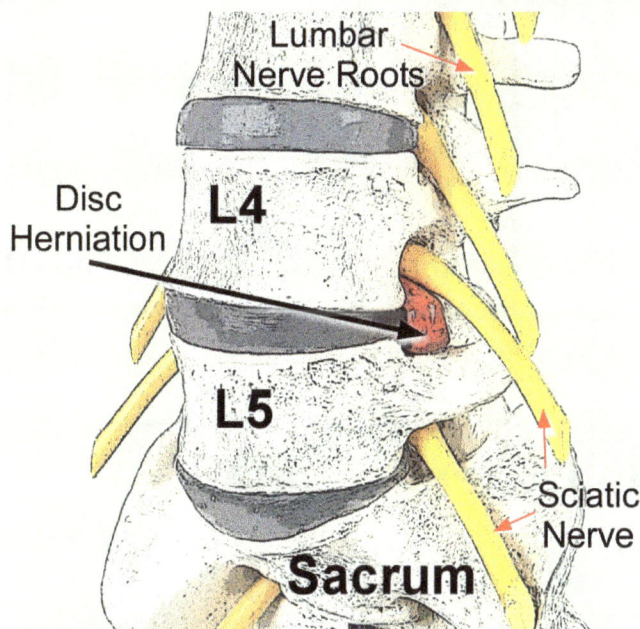

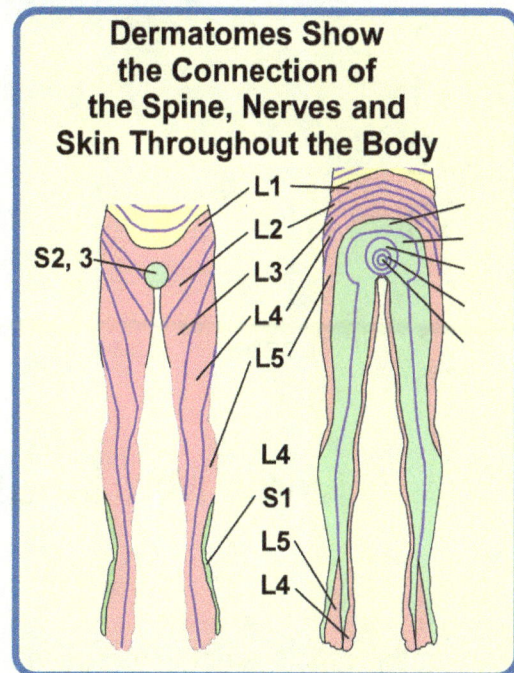

Lumbar Nerve Roots

Disc Herniation

L4

L5

Sacrum

Sciatic Nerve

Dermatomes Show the Connection of the Spine, Nerves and Skin Throughout the Body

L1
L2
L3
L4
L5

S2, 3

L4
S1
L5
L4

## www.MindandBodyExercises.com

I am not a doctor nor claim to be. However, I have a different health, fitness and well-being background spanning almost 40 years. Starting martial training at the age of 16, I have continued training, studying and teaching ever since. Traditional Chinese medicine and qigong can also be studied within some martial arts lineages, which I have pursued. Martial arts are deeply connected to fitness and health, aside from the obvious self-defense benefits. My fellow instructors (and students) and I were taught that it was easier but not ethical to injure someone unless justified. More honorable was to heal injuries or train and teach to not become injured.

# Sciatica - Connection of Pain & Numbness

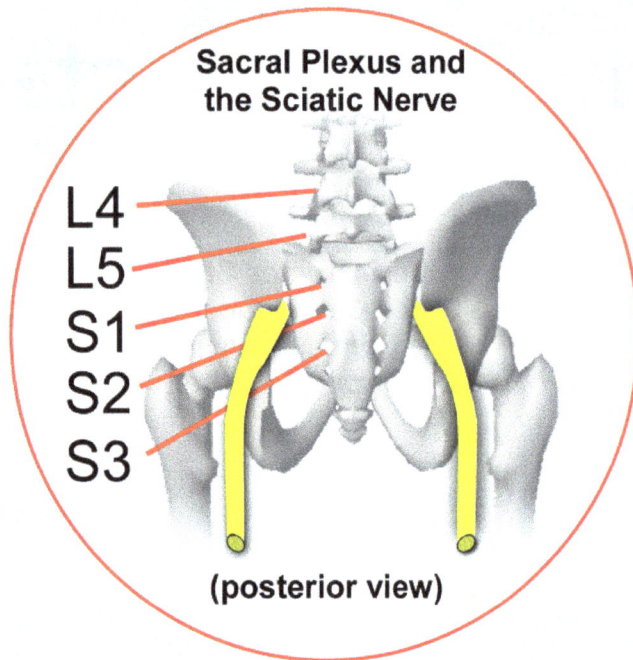

Sacral Plexus and the Sciatic Nerve

L4
L5
S1
S2
S3

(posterior view)

### Nerve Root Issues

| | L4 | L5 | S1 |
|---|---|---|---|
| Pain | | | |
| Numbness | | | |

## www.MindandBodyExercises.com

The point of this article is not to dissuade anyone from gaining medical treatment. But rather encourage the acquiring of information and learning what one's options are before committing to a surgical procedure that may or might not improve your current situation. There is always a risk of having a worse set of circumstances after the procedure. There is not much loss nor risk of trying non-impact exercises, other than one's time and effort. If the exercises don't produce the desired results of pain reduction and back stability, one can always elect to have the surgical procedure afterwards, which will undoubtedly require pain meds, physical therapy and exercises after surgery anyway. *Pay now or pay later* - another term often used in the healthcare industry.

Try to match your body position similar to those as shown. Don't be discouraged by not being able to achieve these stretches but rather do what your body is capable of. Stretches can be performed on the floor, on a mattress or even in a swimming pool or hot tub. Try for a few seconds in each position for a total of a few minutes. As your flexibility increases in the hamstrings, less tension will be placed on the lower back muscles. Try to do some of the exercises everyday for at least a few days in a row. As the pain is relieved, try to add more time for each exercise working up to a total of a half-hour or full hour. As less pain is present, try to maintain a regular schedule of performing these exercises to keep the problem from reoccurring. All stretches should be performed on both sides. Relax the body into the positions in spite of any tension in the muscles. Deep and relaxed breathing (qigong) is essential while performing these exercises.

A key concept in relieving pain is to increase flexibility (range of motion) while building strength, to provide stability and support in the injured areas.

**Piriformis stretch**

Lay flat on the back as bending both knees. Try to cross the right foot over the left knee. Pull the left leg towards your face as the right hip stretches.

**Cat Tilt**

Side View | Top View

Rest on hands and knees as pulling stomach and lower back upwards while pulling chin in towards the chest.

**Torso twist**

Sit on the buttocks with one leg straight and one leg bent and crossed over the other. Turn the upper body opposite while relaxing the back.

**Seated toe touch**

Sit on the buttocks as leaning the upper body forward. Focus more on the torso coming forward than the hands reaching the feet.

**Knee to opposite hand**

Lay flat on your back, bring a bent knee across the other straight leg. Relax the neck and arms as you feel the lower back stretch to the side.

**Bridge (basic)**

Side View | Top View

Lay flat on the back, push hips upward as keeping shoulders and feet on the ground.

**Cobra**

Side View | Top View

Lay flat on the stomach while pushing the hands downward and the head and shoulders upward.

**Dog Tilt**

Side View | Top View

Rest on hands and knees as pulling stomach and lower back downwards while pulling chin upwards.

Side View | Angled View

Can be held for intervals of time at different angles of height or continuously stretching as bending forward.

The above exercises are a sample of various yoga and qigong types of movements that can offer relief of pain for some individuals. Again, it is imperative that the individual becomes educated and aware of what their particular situation is and what movements will help or hinder their body.

_____

**How Deep Breathing Affects Your Health**

Deep breathing is a key component to having a long and healthy life. Through focused and deliberate breathing methods, many positive mental and physical benefits can be achieved.

The average person breathes 12-18 breaths per minute (BPM) during regular activity of standing, sitting & walking, engaging in the sympathetic nervous system (SNS). Constant duration in the SNS dumps neurotransmitters of cortisol and norepinephrine into the blood stream putting the vital organs in a state of constant high alert and stress. Health and fitness experts suggest that 6 BPM is optimal for the lungs to properly oxygenate the whole body, balance the blood chemistry and also remove toxins. The lungs are responsible for removing 70% of the body's waste by-products through exhalation. This is more easily accomplished through mindful breathing patterns from exercises such as mediation, qigong, tai chi and yoga.

**Most people breathe too shallow and too quickly!**

Much recent research has linked stress to poor breathing habits and consequently many ailments. Many modern chronic conditions can be traced back to insufficient cell oxygenation otherwise known as cell hypoxia.

Breathing is one of the few bodily rhythms that we can consciously adjust, along with sleep and elimination. All of these rhythms directly affect our body's delicate blood chemistry. However, our breath is the root power in bringing oxygen (qi) into our body to nourish it down to the cellular level.

Faster breathing is necessary when experiencing truly stressful situations, like being chased by an animal, running from a fire or similar life-threatening situations. However, continued breathing at this pace for an extended period of time puts accumulative stress on all of the body's systems.

The following link has more information from the US National Library of Medicine, National Institutes of Health, that goes a bit deeper into the science of why lower breaths per minute (BPM) is so beneficial.

https://www.ncbi.nlm.nih.gov/pmc/articles/PMC5709795/

# Changing Your Breathing Rhythm

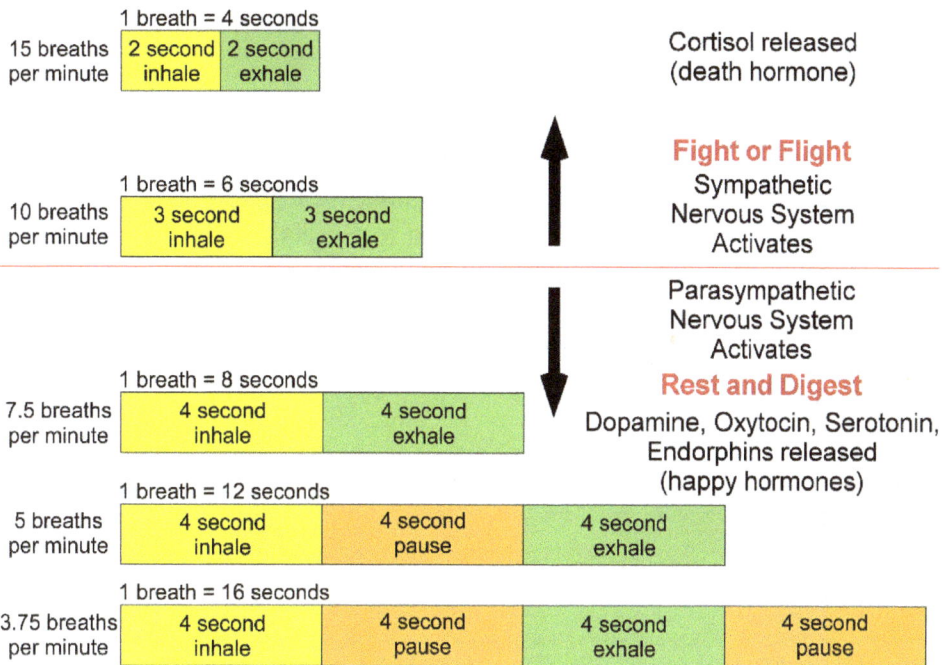

| | | |
|---|---|---|
| 15 breaths per minute | **1 breath = 4 seconds** | Cortisol released (death hormone) |
| | 2 second inhale / 2 second exhale | |

**↑**

**Fight or Flight**
Sympathetic Nervous System Activates

| | |
|---|---|
| 10 breaths per minute | **1 breath = 6 seconds** |
| | 3 second inhale / 3 second exhale |

**↓**

Parasympathetic Nervous System Activates

**Rest and Digest**
Dopamine, Oxytocin, Serotonin, Endorphins released (happy hormones)

| | |
|---|---|
| 7.5 breaths per minute | **1 breath = 8 seconds** |
| | 4 second inhale / 4 second exhale |

| | |
|---|---|
| 5 breaths per minute | **1 breath = 12 seconds** |
| | 4 second inhale / 4 second pause / 4 second exhale |

| | |
|---|---|
| 3.75 breaths per minute | **1 breath = 16 seconds** |
| | 4 second inhale / 4 second pause / 4 second exhale / 4 second pause |

www.MindandBodyExercises.com

# Breathing Patterns

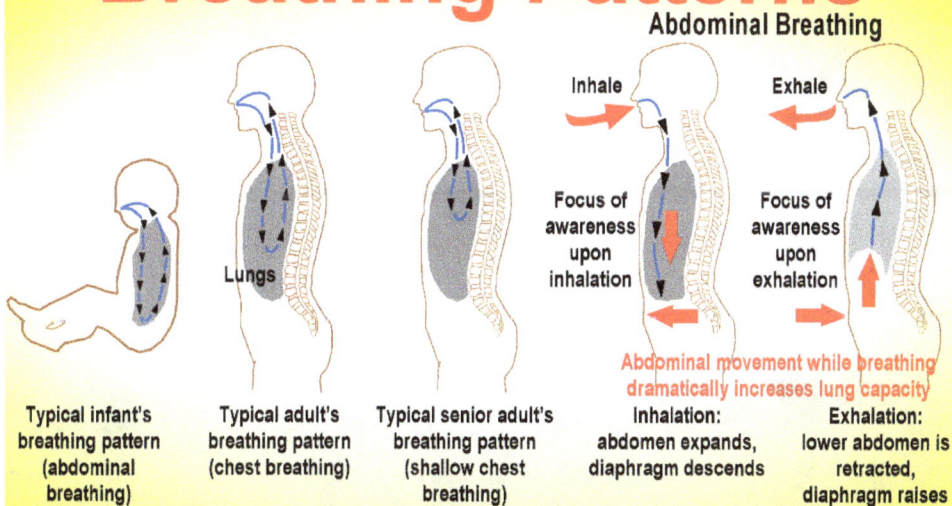

**Abdominal Breathing**

Inhale          Exhale

Focus of awareness upon inhalation

Focus of awareness upon exhalation

Lungs

Abdominal movement while breathing dramatically increases lung capacity

**Typical infant's breathing pattern (abdominal breathing)**

**Typical adult's breathing pattern (chest breathing)**

**Typical senior adult's breathing pattern (shallow chest breathing)**

**Inhalation:** abdomen expands, diaphragm descends

**Exhalation:** lower abdomen is retracted, diaphragm raises

**Deeper breathing is a key component to having a long and healthy life. Through focused and deliberate breathing methods, many positive mental and physical benefits can be achieved.**
www.MindandBodyExercises.com

110

# Specific Methods of Mind-Body Practice

## BaguaZhang

### BaguaZhang (8 Trigram Palm)

*Bagua, Baguazhang, Bagwa, Pakua,* Walking Meditation or "walking of the circle" are all names for this style of Kung Fu training. Translated to English is "8 trigram palm". Bagua is an internal developing style similar to Tai chi and Hsing Yi. Tai chi is often considered to be the softest, Bagua somewhat harder and Hsing Yi the hardest style of the three main internal styles. Hard and soft refer to the control applied to the various movements practiced. Bagua develops stability in motion amongst many other things. *Cheng, Chung, Emei, Sun* are all styles of Baguazhang.

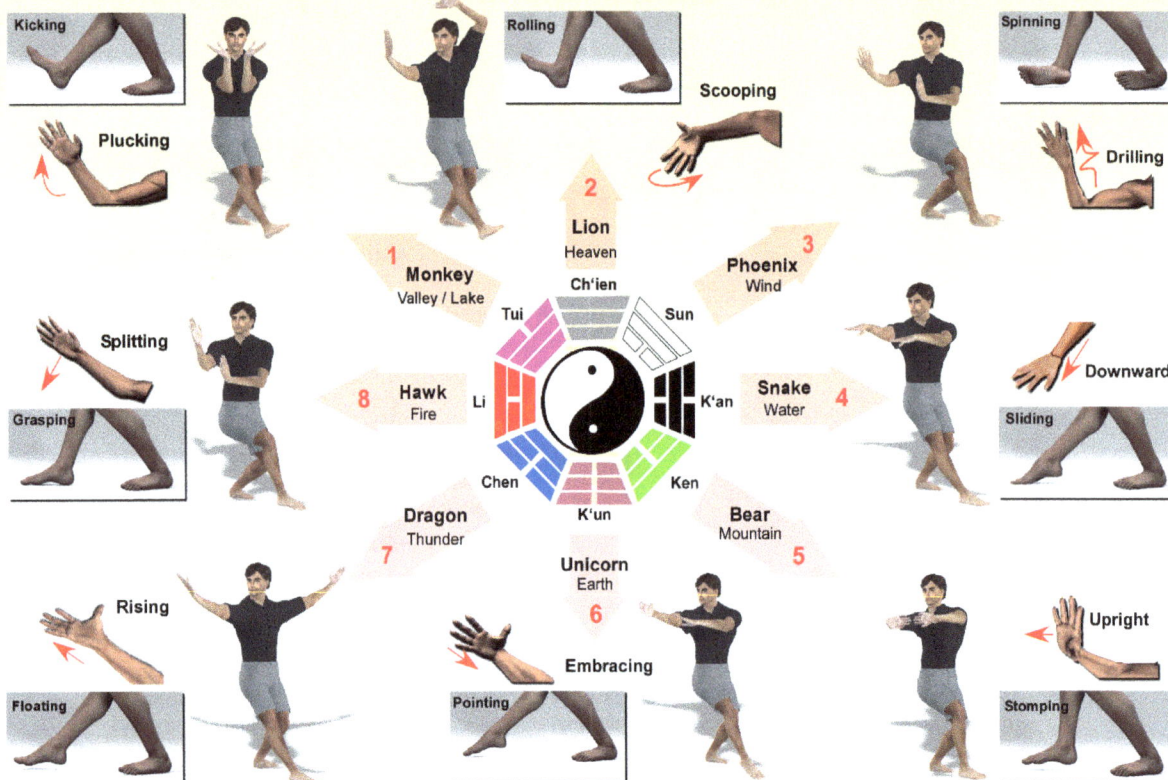

**BaguaZhang (Pakua, moving meditation, circle walking)**     www.MindandBodyExercises.com

**8 Animal Characteristics**     **8 Fundamental Palms**     **8 Stepping Methods**

Deep mindful breathing, specific muscle stretching and deliberate walking techniques are the basis of BagauZhang exercises. Practicing BaguaZhang or Bagua, stepping positions, body postures and changes (transitional stretching movements) enables one to move your body like a spring, being flexible and light but having a lot of strength and power behind the movement. This would be similar to moving as light and smooth as a feather but having the strength and speed of a bear. Attaining certain body alignments within postures, holding that position and moving from one to another is essential to develop overall strength, coordination, balance and increase of energy flow throughout the body. Proper breathing is important in the development of internal strength and has to be in tune with each movement.

Benefits include:

- Calming of the mind

- Focused thought

- Strengthens and relaxes muscles

- Can be practices as "Moving Meditation"

- Attention to body alignments

- Cultivates internal energy (qi)

- Develops the physical body from the inside out

- Slow, medium & fast body motions

- Static (isometric) as well as continuous (isotonic) movements

Deep mindful breathing, specific muscle stretching and deliberate walking techniques are the basis of BaguaZhang exercises. Practicing BaguaZhang or Bagua, stepping positions, body postures and changes (transitional stretching movements) enables one to move your body like a spring, being flexible and light but having a lot of strength and power behind the movement. This would be similar to moving as light and smooth as a feather but having the strength and speed of a bear.

Attaining certain body alignments within postures, holding that position and moving from one to another is essential to develop overall strength, coordination, balance and increase of energy flow throughout the body. Proper breathing is important in the development of internal strength and has to be in tune with each movement. These postures can be practiced as static exercises for any length of time (typically 20 seconds to 5 minutes or more), or dynamically while performing the different stepping methods.

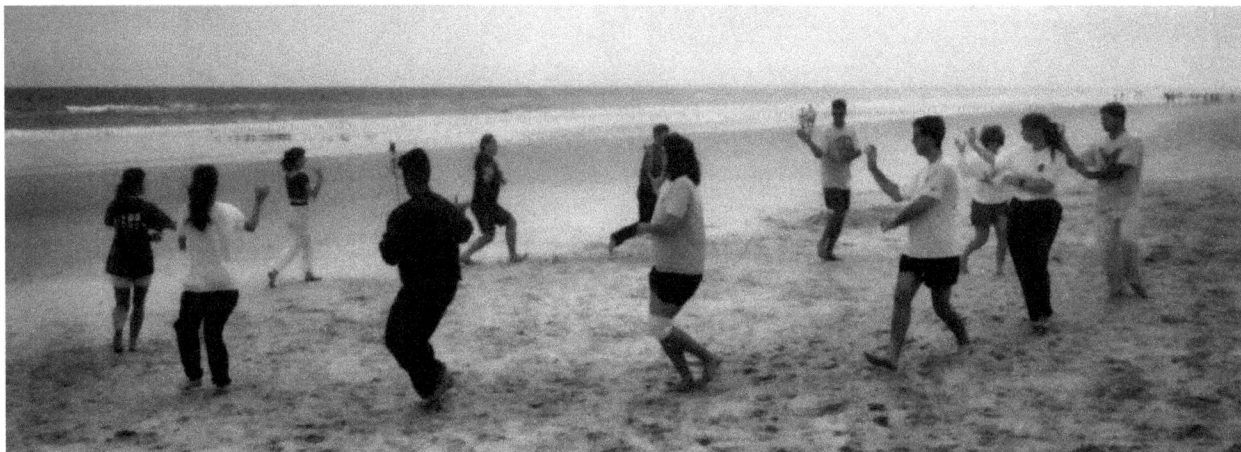

**"Workout"** is to exercise to stay healthy with no specific goals.

**"Training"** is what some do, for a specific goal or performance. Sometimes training is to increase knowledge of a particular skill set.

**"Practice**" is what individuals commit to do, in order to improve, increase or perfect their skills for a specific goal, performance or mastery.

BaguaZhang is an exercise method that can be a workout, training or practice depending upon the goals of the individual.

BaguaZhang exercises consist of:
- gentle stretching
- deep rhythmic breathing
- walking exercises for the lower body and blood circulation
- exercises that have been time-proven over hundreds of years

BaguaZhang translates to "8 Trigram Palm."

The Bagua is an 8-sided shape which can represent harmony and balance. Trigrams are relative to Chinese philosophy from the I-Ching, which has been studied by millions for hundreds of years to learn to exist within balance.

https://youtu.be/sKEpWtwEpVk

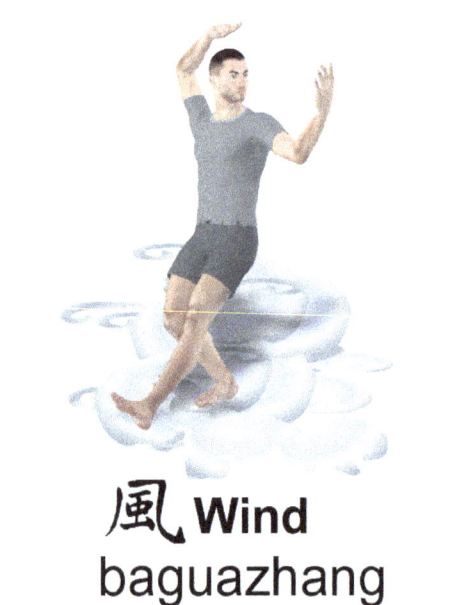

風 **Wind**
baguazhang

# Meditation

## Why Practice Meditation?

My definition of meditation is practices where an individual trains their mind to achieve a mode of consciousness to realize benefits. Meditation does not necessarily need to be done in a lotus position nor, hours of sitting motionless. However, these are methods of meditation. So can walking, gardening, playing an instrument, drawing, painting, journaling, yoga, tai chi, qigong, archery, target shooting and many other methods can be used as meditative practices.

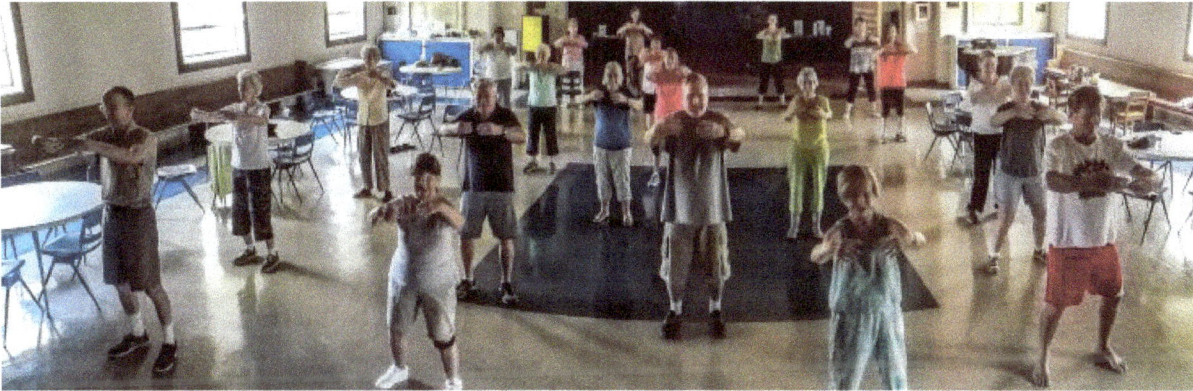

I may have had some second thoughts or skepticism when I first started to learn of meditation practices. However, I was 16 years old at the time and had very little life experience and not much wisdom at this point in my life. Eastern philosophy and meditation practices from martial arts, qigong, yoga and others were not widely accepted in the United States in the early 80's and definitely not in Midwest suburbia of the Chicago area of Illinois. Martial arts schools at this time in the US were looked upon as being religious, cult-like, or at the very least a cultural-shock to my conservative upbringing.

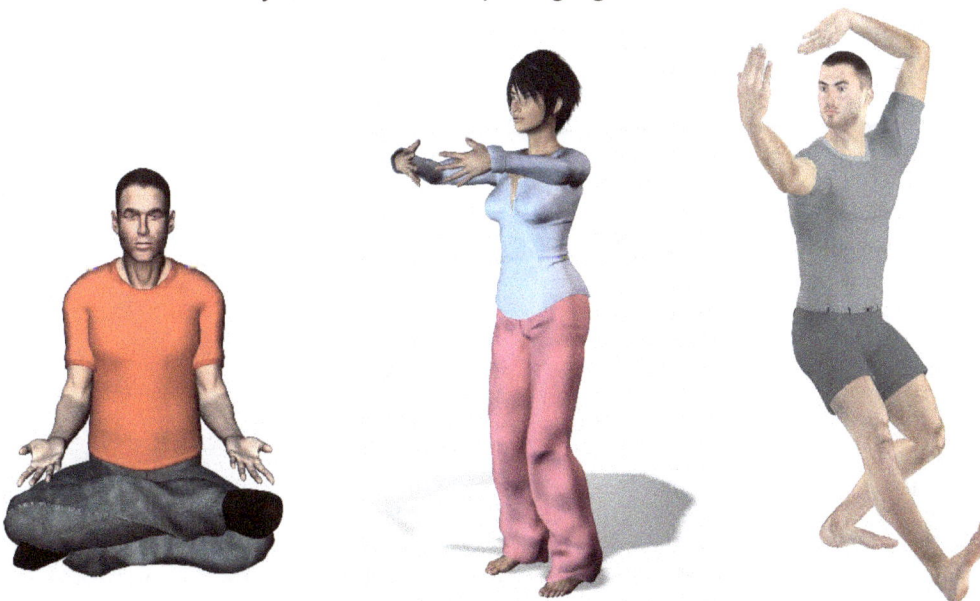

When we are young, we can often be more influenced and possibly manipulated by others in order to see their viewpoints or beliefs in their personal agenda. I may have experienced some of these issues to some extent. However, in my case this turned out to not be a bad thing but rather a life-changing event that allowed me to gain benefits from meditation for decades forward.

> "You should sit in meditation for twenty minutes every day unless you're too busy Then you should sit for an hour."
>
> - Old Zen saying

Whatever reluctance I held at the time for these methods, soon diminished as I was able to see and feel the benefits of my training, while I saw my elders and peers' health and well-being suffer from years of unregulated emotional stress and physical tension.

## SIMPLE MEDITATION.

Sit comfortably. Breathe naturally. Tune into your breath, follow the sensation of inhaling from your nose to abdomen and out again. Let tension go with each exhalation. When you notice your mind wandering, return to your breath.

## THE BENEFITS OF MEDITATION

Inreases Immunity

Emotional Balance

Lowers Blood Pressure

Calmness

Increases creativity

Decreases muscle tension

Helps with weight loss

Relief from asthma

Relaxes nervous system

Builds self confidence

Increases serotonin

Meditation practices can offer so much in relation to cultivating the mind, body and spiritual harmony that many seek to achieve but really have no plan, method or goal as to where meditation can guide them to. I have been able to build and nurture (cultivate) a relationship with my mental thought process, my physical being and my spiritual awareness of something bigger and more profound than the mundane life we often possess and accept.

Meditation has offered me so much. Specifically, on the mental level I have been able to release mental stress and achieve consistent focus and clarity. On the physical level I have learned to be able to recognize and release muscular tension by slowing my breath rate, heart rate and blood pressure. On the spiritual level I have been able to enter into a deeper sense of self-awareness and realization that our life is a series of lessons to be learned to hopefully serve a greater purpose. We can find religious or spiritual leaders to help guide us through this journey. Or we can venture inward and go direct to the source if this is where we choose to put our efforts. Meditation is not a replacement for one's faith but rather a way to enhance and understand it. Meditation is a tool to be used for the benefit of the practitioner. Based upon these concepts, I feel that my meditation practices have much more to offer me in my next stages of life.

**NO MEMBERSHIP NECESSARY**

**NO EQUIPMENT REQUIRED**

**NO GURU NEEDED**

**PRACTICE ANYWHERE, ANYTIME**

**UNCOMPLICATED**

**FREE**

There needs to be a mental intention behind whatever practice one chooses to pursue. Sometimes people get so hung up with just the word of "meditation" and thinking that to meditate one needs to become more spiritual, metaphysical or adopt some form of religion. I have taught literally hundreds of tai chi and qigong classes where at the end I explain about it being a moving meditation as well as vipassana and body scan meditation all in one. Occasionally, someone will be quite shocked and state something like "I didn't know this was a religion; I am not interested in changing or doing your religion." It is pretty hard to try to convince someone at this point, being that they felt great while doing the exercises. However, due to some narrow-mindedness or lack of knowledge on the subject, they now feel indifferent towards the techniques. For those still open to learning, I will ask how many enjoy cooking, walking, photography, listening to music, gardening, etc. seeing that these can all be used as various forms of creative or moving meditation. Meditation is not a religion but rather a method to become more self-aware.

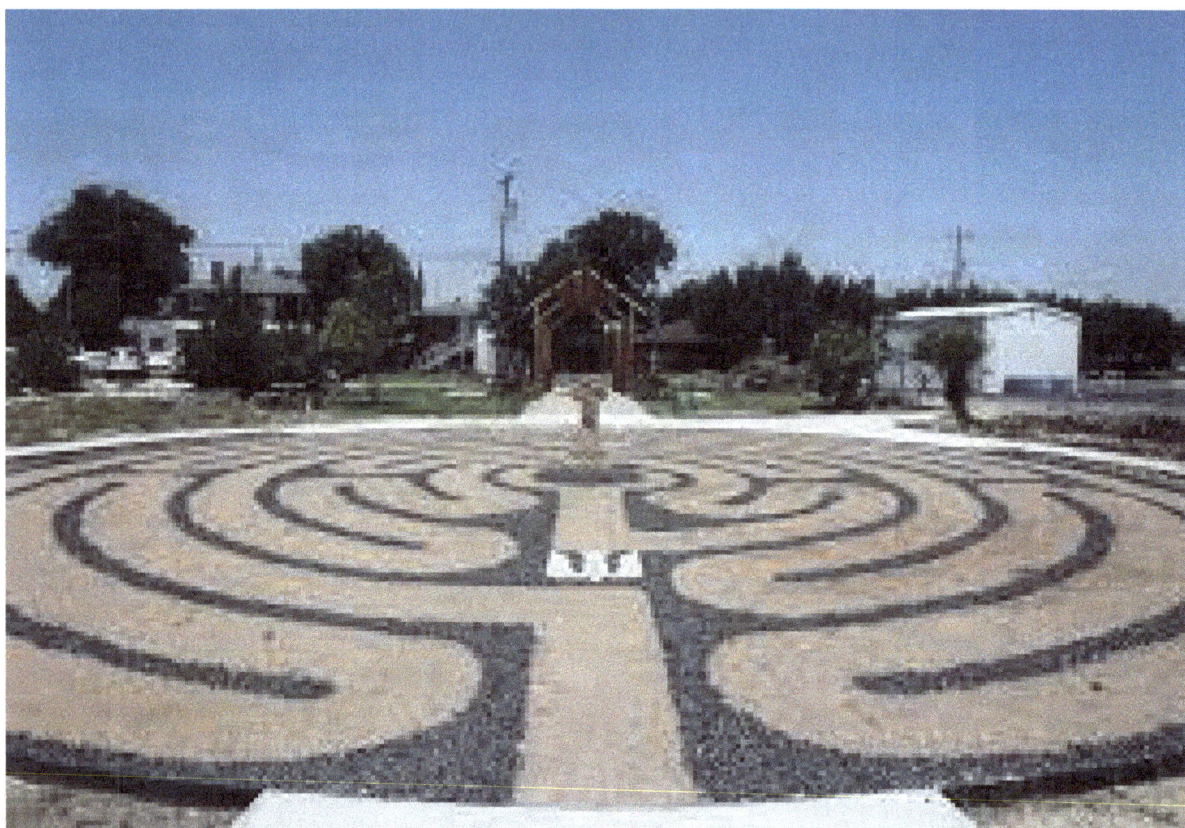

Creative meditation requires alert and active engagement of the consciousness, often with the goal of providing an environment for an inner dialogue within one's thoughts as opposed to a passive acceptance of whatever thoughts may arise. Creative practices often have a physical element involved that links the body and mind together, such as sketching, journaling, gardening, tai chi, yoga, and others.

This is somewhat different from methods like vipassana or loving kindness meditation methods, where the inner dialogue is mostly isolated from physical movements or engagements. On the other hand, creative meditation can be similar to drumming or ritual body postures in that the practitioner still needs to have an awareness of their physical being holding its space in the 3-dimensional world whether holding a yoga-like posture or a paintbrush in hand.

Another form of creative meditation that I have encountered is that of calligraphy qigong. Qigong is roughly translated to "breath work" and calligraphy is a visual art form of writing. When qigong and calligraphy are combined, practitioners develop their own qi (energy or lifeforce) resources by receiving, circulating, and storing qi while performing each brush stroke of a particular pictogram.

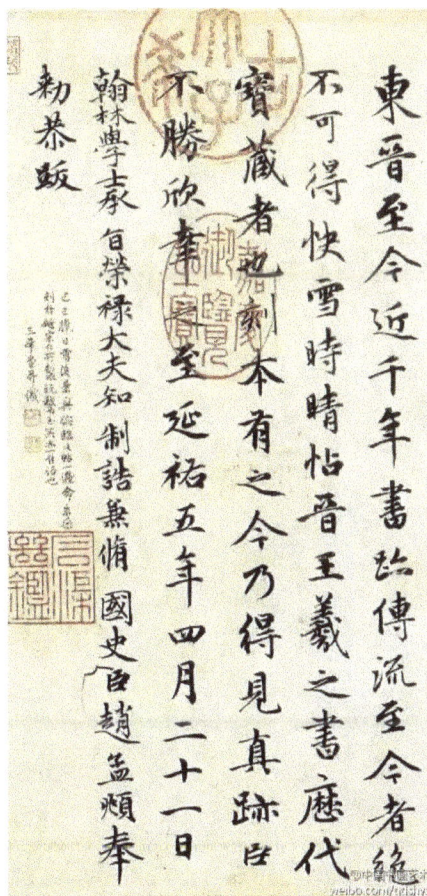

From my own experiences, all of these practices are neither good nor bad, nor absolute but rather fluid and able to be adjusted to an individual's goals, perspectives and perhaps the mindset towards particular practices. Similarly, to the chef in the kitchen, who can make whatever meal they care to produce because they are in charge of all of their tools and ingredients within their cooking space, the meditator can pick and choose what suits their objectives.

## Insight Meditation (Vipassana)

*You should sit in meditation for twenty minutes every day unless you're too busy. Then you should sit for an hour."* Or *"If you have time to breathe, you have time to meditate."* These are great quotes to ponder but regardless, meditation is an active practice that will not happen if I (we) do not make it happen.

I think many people confuse religion with philosophy. My understanding of religion is that it is a belief system based upon faith or what cannot be seen. Whereas philosophy is generally a rational investigation of truths. With this being said, I don't think I would even enter into the conversation of how meditation is not religion, but rather a tool that could enhance one's religious beliefs or other aspects of their life, unless they had an openness to begin with. I have found that trying to convince someone of something usually doesn't achieve the desired results.

Insight meditation is also known as Vipassana and is known to be the oldest of Buddhist meditation practices coming directly from the *Satipatthana* Sutta which is the "Discourse on the Establishing of Awareness" attributed to the Buddha himself. Vipassana meditation is a direct but gradual training of self-awareness or mindfulness usually over a period of years. During practice, a student's attention is focused inward towards an intense contemplation of particular aspects of one's existence. The meditator trains to be more and more self-aware of their own flowing life experience.

## What Happpens When You Hold Your Breath For A Few Minutes A Day?
### The Benefits Of Intermittent Hypoxia

**Benefits:**
1. Vasodilation & Improved Circulation
2. Increase In Red Blood Cells
3. Memory & Cognitive Function
4. Induces Cancer Protecting Protein p53
5. Proliferates Antiaging Stem Cells

**Methods:**
1. Rechaka Pranayama
2. Wim Hof Method
3. Buteyko Method
4. Hypoxia Therapy
5. Altitude Training

**May Treat:**
1. Alzheimer's, Dementia, Parkinson's
2. Type 2 Diabetes
3. Coronary Artery Disease
4. Osteoarthritis
5. Inflammation
6. Autoimmune Conditions
7. Depression

Fact: Russian scientists have used intermittent hypoxia as 'hypoxia therapy' to treat a variety of health issues for several decades.

visit: TheRenegadePharmacist.com/breathhold for the full article and citations.

**RENEGADE PHARMACIST** TRUTH PRESCRIBED

https://therenegadepharmacist.com/what-happens-when-you-hold-your-breath-for-a-few-minutes-a-day-the-benefits-of-intermittent-hypoxia-rechaka-kumbhaka-buteyko-the-wim-hof-method/

Put aside time on your schedule to practice Vipassana meditation. Find a quiet room or space within or near your home. Sit upright but comfortably and relaxed in a sturdy chair. Relax and close your eyes. Make your breathing deeper and longer with a 4-second pause between each inhale an exhale. Move your attention away from your breathing and onto other observations of your thoughts. Relax your neck and shoulders and work your way down your torso using just enough muscular tension to hold your body upright. Experience going through a progression from physical awareness to mental awareness and then to an emotional release to become present in the moment. Once you are comfortable with the physical awareness of your body, move on to becoming aware of your senses and what is occurring in your immediate environment inside and out. Listen closely to maybe hear the A/C or heater turning off, bringing your focus maybe to the refrigerator now humming away in the background of your awareness. Each time a distraction presents itself, acknowledge it and then become aware of the next sound. If there is no sound, move onto feeling the touch of your body in the chair or your feet on the floor. Then another thought will appear, like how long have I been sitting here, whether the room is warm, or what time of day is it? All trivial thoughts within your inner dialogue that you can continue to acknowledge and then let fade away. Slowly open your eyes to the room, appearing slightly brighter and sharper. You will feel refreshed and calm thereafter.

The Maharishi Mahesh Yogi (1917-2008) is known to have founded Transcendental Meditation or simply TM, inspired from his teacher and guru Swami Brahmananda Saraswati (who died 1953), and drawing upon the ancient Indian traditions of Vedic. He introduced the technique to the United States in the 1960s, where the British rock band the Beatles and other celebrities embraced the teachings adding to its popularity.

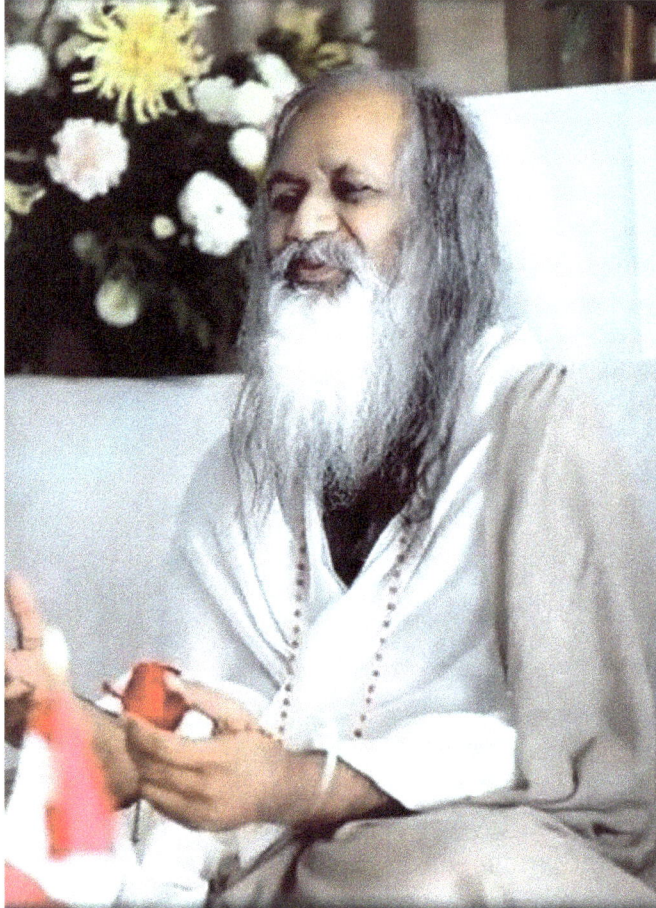

Maharishi Mahesh Yogi

Transcendental Meditation is a meditation method that attempts to avoid distracting thoughts while promoting a state of relaxed awareness. Somewhat different from other types of meditation methods, TM teaches practitioners to stay focused on a mantra which is a specific phrase. The mantra is then repeated internally within one's inner dialogue of their thoughts. Transcendental Meditation came to be taught and practiced as a non-spiritual nor religious path toward mental, emotional, and physical well-being.

The goal when meditating, is to "transcend" the regular thought process. It is replaced by a state of pure consciousness. In this state, the practitioner seeks to achieve perfect stillness, rest, order, and stability, completely without mental boundaries. This state of being is thought to lead to increased contentment, creativity and vitality.

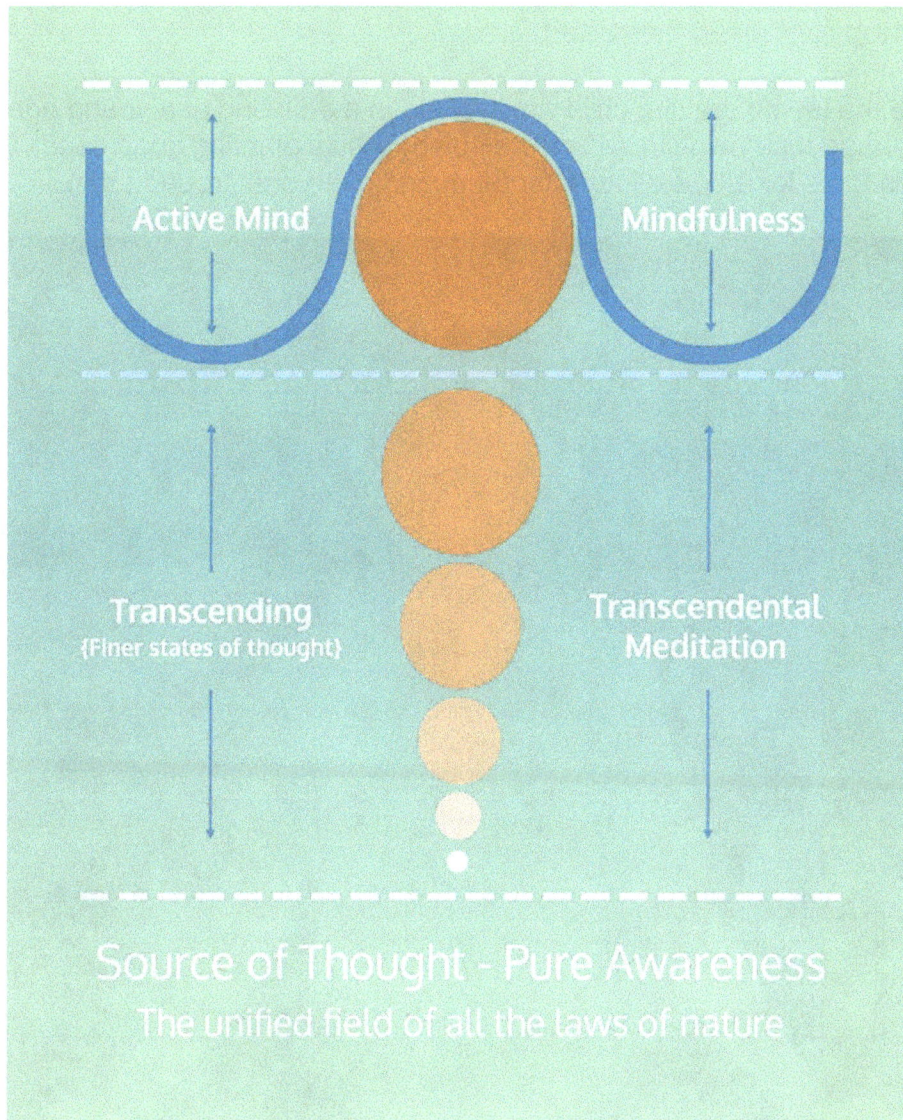

**Active Mind** — **Mindfulness**

**Transcending**
(Finer states of thought)

**Transcendental Meditation**

**Source of Thought - Pure Awareness**
The unified field of all the laws of nature

From a physiological perspective, Transcendental Meditation can relax and revitalize the body and the mind by engaging in the parasympathetic nervous system where stress and anxiety are reduced, blood pressure (hypertension) decreases, and changing the blood chemistry to help relieve depression.

A typical TM practice session might follow this progression:
- Sit in a comfortable chair keeping the feet on the ground and hands in your lap. Legs and arms are uncrossed.
  - Eyes are closed while taking a few deep breaths in order to relax the body.
  - Repeat a mantra in your mind.
  - When you recognize you're having a thought, return to the mantra.
  - After about 20 minutes, begin to move your fingers and toes, easing yourself back to the world.
  - Open your eyes.
  - Sit and relax for a few more minutes until ready to continue with your day

I especially like the idea of getting children involved in meditating at a young age. Teaching kids how to manage their own stress and well-being is like planting good seeds with the intent of a giving them tools for a better future for them and everyone around them.

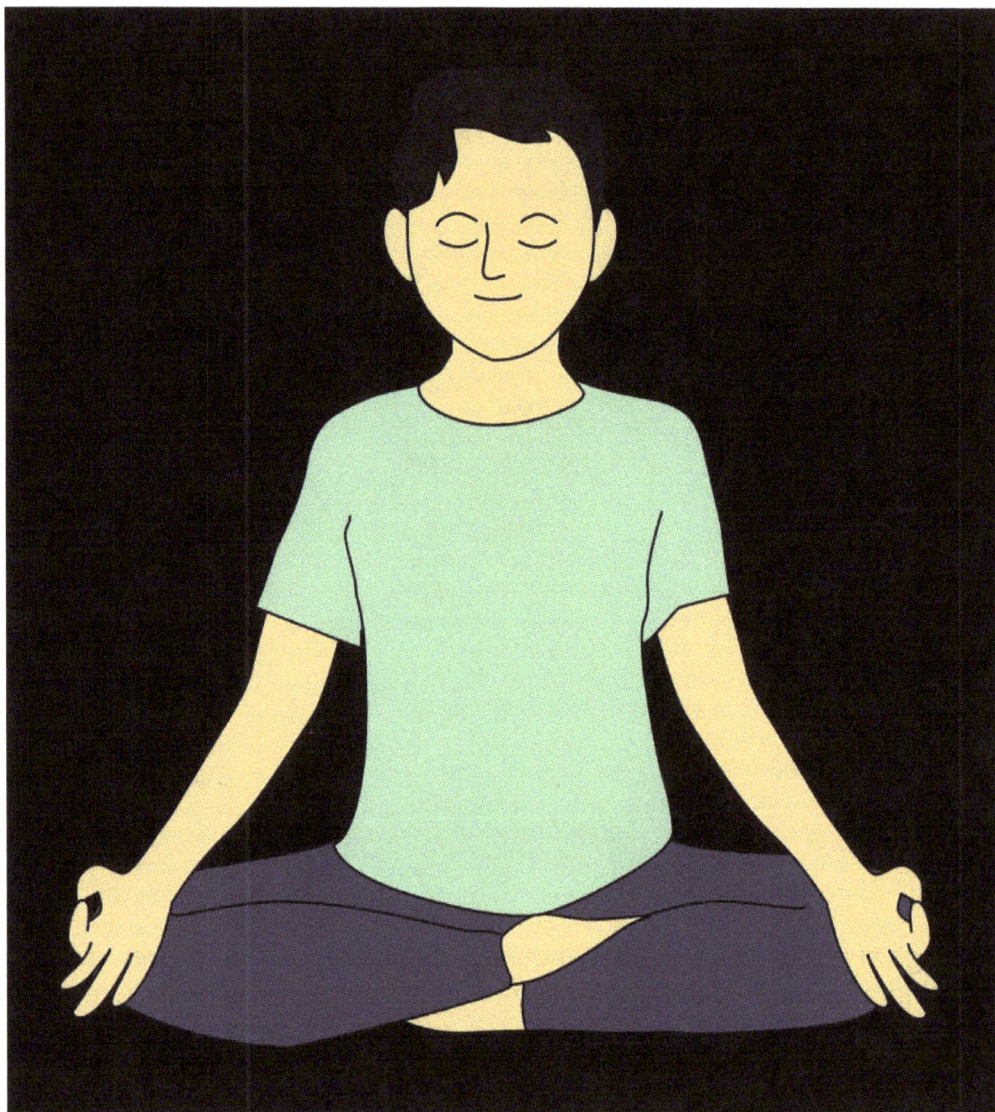

I researched that in China, children do meditate at the different age levels in school. It is also different in different schools. In some elementary schools, kids might meditate every day. In middle school they might twice a week. In some high schools, they might meditate once a week. I did find also, that in a particular primary school in Foshan, China, parents objected to meditation practices in place of nap time at school. The school was basically forced to remove the practice from the school setting. Maybe things in China are more like the US than we care to admit. Regardless, mediation practices have been part of many cultures for thousands of years.

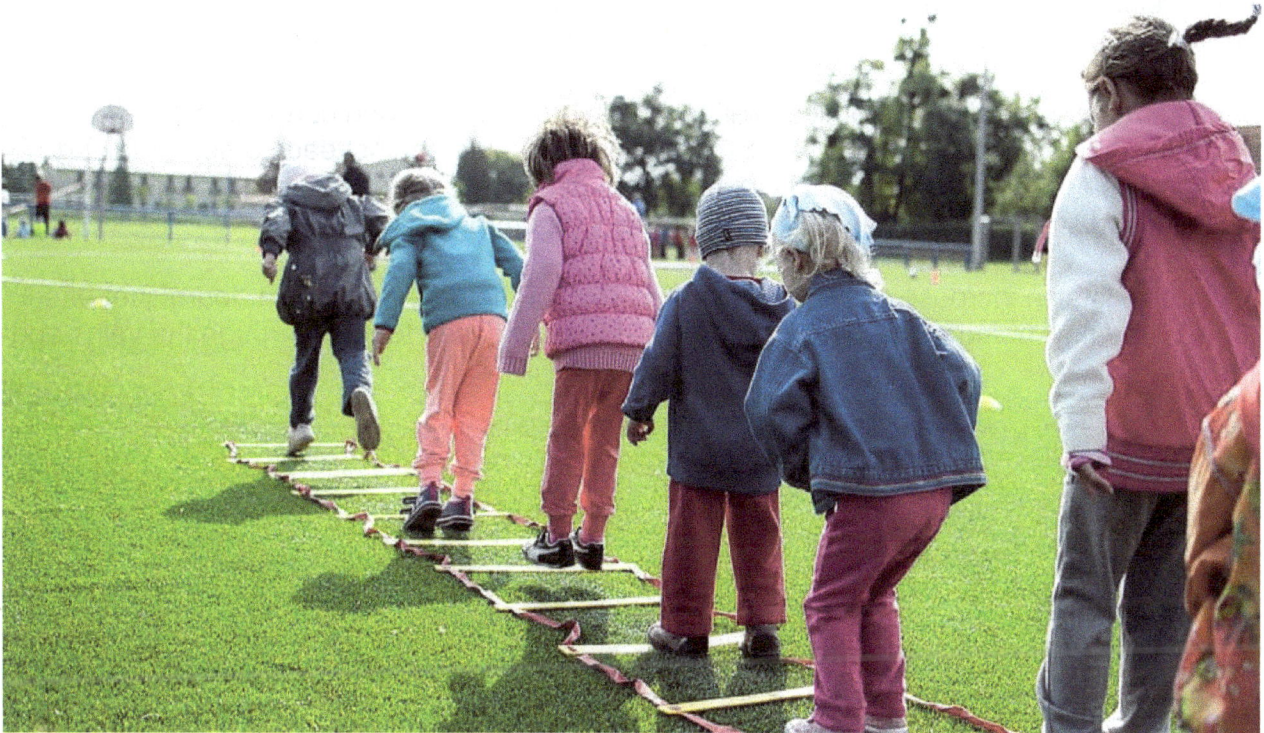

Let us not forget that in years past, recess and physical education (PE) were part of the school day from kindergarten through elementary school. High school students had PE every school day until graduation. **Regular exercise has been known and proven to help manage stress and maintain better health and mental well-being.** Meditation is a mental exercise that can be accomplished in many ways. Aside from the still of sitting meditation that most people think of, there are also moving mediation methods such as walking, tai chi, yoga and qigong. Gardening can even be a type of mediation as some grade schools get the kids outdoors and get their hands in the dirt.

Remember, unhealthy kids quickly turn into unhealthy adults. The health of our people is directly affecting the safety of our nation. For the sake of our youth and ultimately our country, we need to implement more PE, meditation of some sort, and health education back into the school system, as a priority and not just a minimal requirement.

Forms or exercise sets are a way to link many various movements into an organized flow or progression from one exercise to the next. This concept is similar to the current trend of "yoga flow" but actually has been practiced for hundreds, if not thousands of years.

Gentle stretching in all 3 anatomical planes (transverse, sagittal and coronal) is a way to directly exercise the organs by making them move and slide against each other, breaking down adhesions. Moving the spinal column in "all directions, every day" is a way to maintain flexibility and strength of the spine and its many components.

Circulation is also increased as the gentle squishing of the core provides a "tourniquet effect" of the blood flow being somewhat restricted and then released to flush through the veins and arteries.

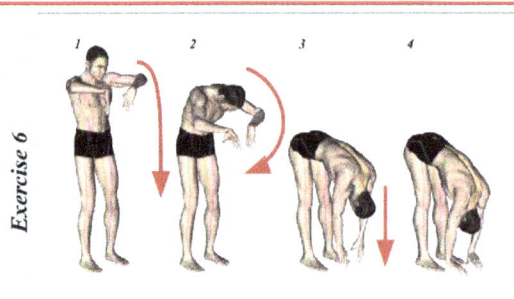

**Exercise 6**

NOTES: *1- hands hang loosely in front of face. 2- chin to the chest as bending one vertebrae at a time while 3- bending downward. 4- Reverse by raising from the lower back, one vertebrae at a time.*

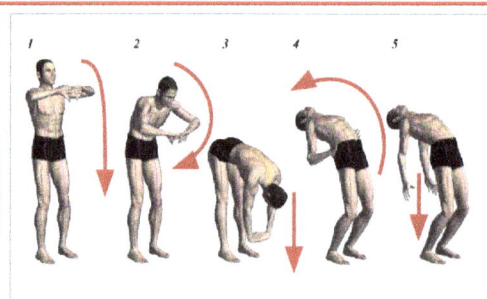

**Exercise 7**

NOTES: *1-3- same as exercise 6 but 4- bending knees as reversing to stand up. 4- hands on lower back/hips while arching backward. 5- extra challenge in letting arms dangle loosely at the sides.*

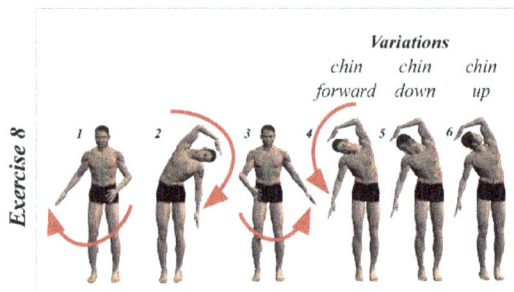

**Exercise 8**

**Variations**

chin forward    chin down    chin up

NOTES: *1- Circle arms to the right and 2- overhead finishing with arms dangling to the side. 3- Reverse & repeat on opposite side. 4-6- Turn chin forward, down & up for variations of the neck stretch.*

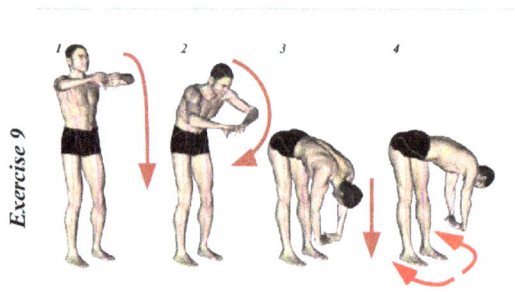

**Exercise 9**

NOTES: *1-3- same as exercise 6 once you are at your lowest point, then 4- gently reaching toward left ankle then back to right ankle. Reverse by raising from the lower back, one vertebrae at a time.*

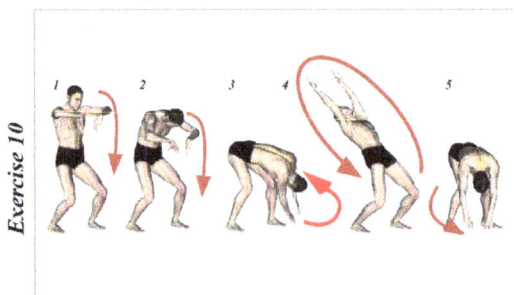

**Exercise 10**

NOTES: *1-3- same as exercise 6 (knees bent) once you are at your lowest point, then 4- gently reaching toward left ankle then lean back to circle torso back to the 5- right ankle. Reverse circle & torso opposite direction to repeat.*

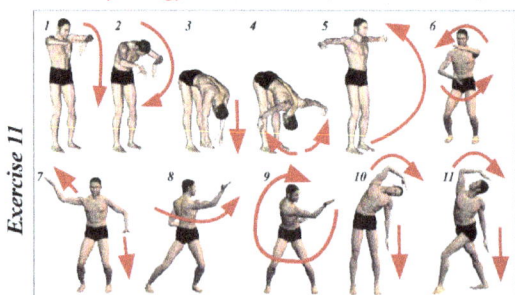

**Exercise 11**

NOTES: *Combination of exercises 6 & 8. 1-3- execute just as ex. 6, to sides. 5- raise back to upright. 6- bend knees as arms make a b arm pushes down. 8- twist torso to left as shifting weight towards le lean sideways from torso as arms dangle overhead & to the side. 1 Repeat again and start opposite side at step 6.*

125

**Top 10 Benefits of Meditation**:
- Reduced Stress.
- Emotional Balance.
- Increased Focus.
- Reduced Pain.
- Reduced Anxiety.
- Increased Creativity.
- Reduced Depression.
- Increased Memory

Carve out time in your schedule to practice a 15-minute body scan meditation practice. You will thank yourself afterwards. Set an alarm for 15 minutes or longer if you care to. As the wise old saying states "if you don't have time to meditate for an hour every day, you should meditate for two hours". We can make time to do the things we prioritize if we care to do so.

Lay flat on a couch or flat comfortable surface allowing yourself to go through a progression from physical awareness to mental realization, and then to an emotional release to become present in the moment. Become aware of your body becoming a bit heavier as you put your focus into your body instead of everything outside of your physical being. From here focus on your breathing becoming deeper and longer with pauses between each inhale and exhale.

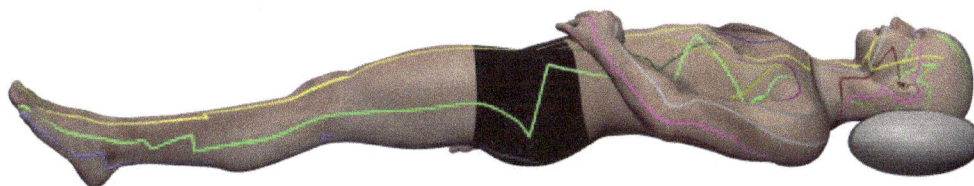

Start at your head and work your way towards your feet. This allows you to release muscular tension as you move downwards ending in your toes and then out and away from your body. Become aware of the tension in your eyelids, eyebrows, jaw, and lips allowing you to relax in these same areas by first tensing and then releasing the muscles.

Feel the tension in your upper back and move your neck and shoulders a little side to side, and up and down to feel the contrast between tension and relaxation of these areas. Stressful emotions of anxiety or frustration develop in your neck and shoulders. Once you direct your focus on these muscle areas, you may be able to engage them with your thoughts to relax them and the surrounding muscle areas.

Work your way down through your torso, letting your skin and muscles hang and sink into the couch beneath you. Your hip bones (pelvis) sink into your glutes. Once you are comfortable with the physical awareness of your body, move on to becoming aware of your senses and what is occurring in your immediate environment. Your fingertips and toe tips may tingle when you focus more on your breathing, all while relaxing of muscular tension throughout your whole body.

When your alarm goes off, open your eyes slowly and re-enter into seeing what you are around. The rest of your body may be more relaxed and comfortable, while feeling calm and refreshed thereafter. The room may appear slightly brighter and sharper. You usually will feel better during and after these practices. Sensations of feeling more refreshed, more calm, more aware, and even more energetic after each session. This session allowed you to "reset" your tension in your body, while releasing mental stress. When your body is relaxed, your emotions become neutral or calm once again.

These practice sessions may become priceless for some people. With these methods, you can have control over your well-being on the levels of physical (body), mental (mind) and emotional (self-awareness). Often, I see people who are constantly seeking the goals of achieving pleasure, peacefulness, joy, love, compassion, ecstasy, and bliss but not being aware that we ourselves are in control of gaining and maintaining these aspects of our lives.

# 8 benefits of meditation found from research studies

1  Meditation can reduce the wake time for people with sleeping problems by up to 50%

2  Practicing meditation for 6-9 months can reduce anxiety by 60%

3  People with back pain were more likely to experience a 30% improvement in their ability to carry out daily tasks compared to those only taking medication

4  Mindfulness meditation can reduce depression relapses by up to 12%

5  People who meditated over an eight-week period changed the expression of 172 genes that regulate inflammation, circadian rhythms, and glucose metabolism

6  Meditation leads to massive increases in regional brain gray matter density

7  Meditation plays a critical role in delaying the onset and slowing the progression of Alzheimer's disease by increasing telomerase enzyme by 43%

8  Meditation may reduce PTSD symptoms 73% of the time

HackSpirit

https://hackspirit.com/25-surprising-meditation-statistics-everyone-needs-to-know/

## Singing Bowls Meditation

A singing bowl or standing bell are mostly crystal or metal alloy bowls where, by rubbing a mallet around the bowl's outer rim and edges produce sounds. Singing bowls and sometimes gongs surround the user with tones that offer the goal of relaxation by decreasing stress, anxiety, and depression. These sounds offer an escape from the everyday incessant inner dialogue or chatter of thoughts within one's mind. Singing bowl techniques can be very mind engaging, similar to meditation practices and yoga, and are often practiced in tandem.

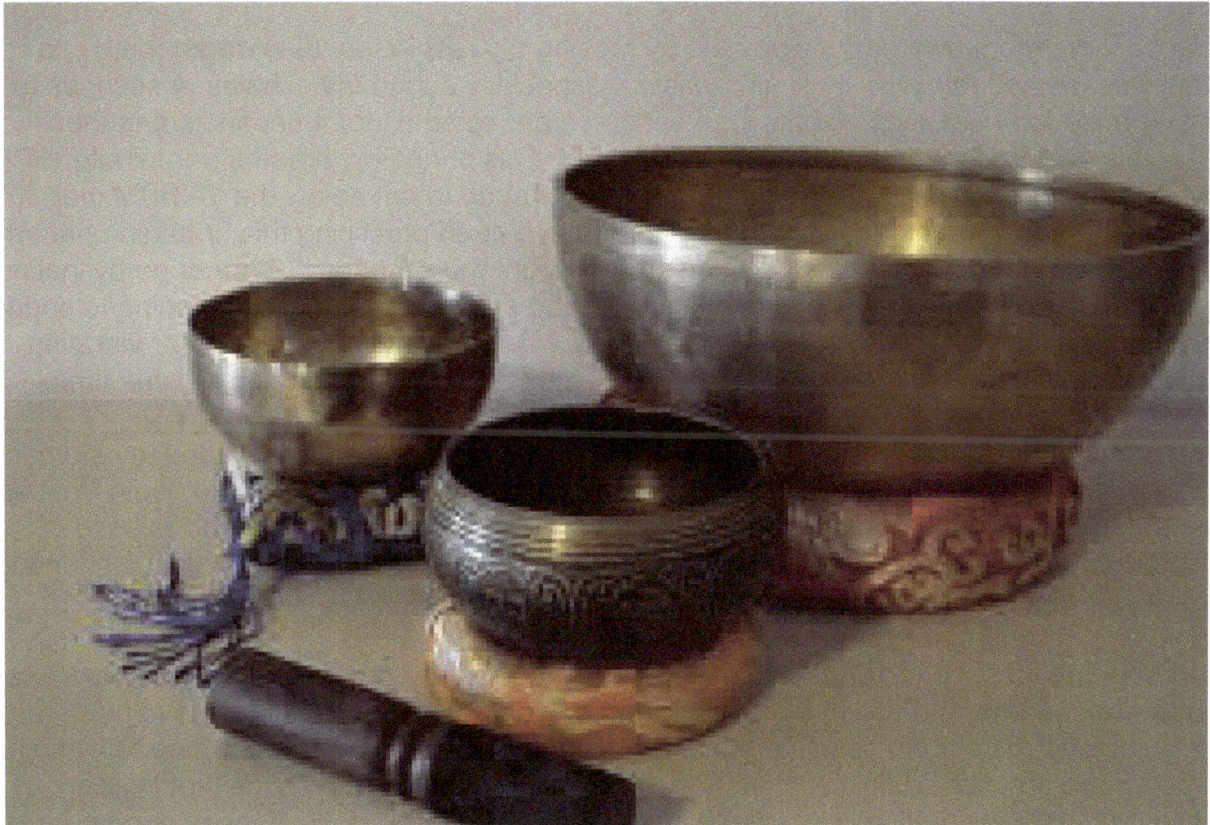

Standing bells historically were a bowl or gong and struck with a wooden or felted mallet. Use goes back thousands of years, with origins in China and Mongolia. Tibetan Buddhist monasteries used the bowls in this manner to keep time or to signal the end of a meditation.

Theories regarding sound bowls claim that specific sounds can calm the mind by entraining the brain's electrical impulses to mimic those found while in states of deep concentration, meditation, or relaxation. Theta waves are present when one is in deep concentration or meditation. From listening to singing bowls, one can guide their mind towards theta brain wave activity.

Click on the link to begin a "A Sound Meditation with Quartz Crystal Bowls".
Once I started the audio file, I took a moment or two to take in the sounds I was hearing. I have practiced other meditation practices using sounds and/or music, so I had an idea of what to expect. This was to be a different "flavor" of a wide palette of meditation techniques.

After a few seconds, I put my focus on my breathing rhythm and body alignments. I find it easier to engage my thoughts by performing a mental inventory of the physical aspects of the meditation practice, kind of a scan from head to toe. I close my eyes lightly while I sit upright, but in a relaxed posture. I also become aware of my head pushing upward as my shoulders relax and sink downward. By gently stretching my neck side to side and forward and backward, I am able to release more tension in my face, neck, upper back and even my shoulders. The sounds continue to change in volume and tones, which is somewhat relaxing to my hearing and consequently, my whole body through my nervous system.

I then become more aware of my breaths by moving my respiratory diaphragm (belly), to further release and relax the muscular tension, especially during my exhales. 4 seconds to inhale, pause for 4 seconds, exhale for 4 seconds, pause again for 4 seconds, and then repeat this sequence with another 4 second inhale. This brings my breaths per minute (BPM) down to just below 4 respirations; more than slow enough to get below the 10 BPM that engages the parasympathetic nervous system. I have been practicing this breathing pattern (box breathing) for decades now, so I don't really count the seconds but rather go by instinct to lengthen my breaths. The sounds continue in the background and are beginning to sound and feel more like vibrations than individual tones. I can feel my body buzzing or vibrating also during this part of the session. It is quite relaxing and comfortable at the same time.

Now I can feel my mouth become moist, my palms and feet become warm, and my stomach begins to gurgle a bit. My brain is telling my body that I am relaxed enough to begin "rest and digest". I become aware of my thoughts and continue the downward scan and release of muscular tension along the way, all the way down to my feet and toes. I maintain just enough tension to maintain my body posture but not too stiff or too relaxed.

Upon finishing I feel calm, refreshed, at ease and clearer. The room is quieter, but now I can hear the refrigerator and A/C in the background. My emotions feel as if they have been reset, for now at least. The room seems brighter, and my eyes focus a bit sharper for a few minutes thereafter the practice. This is a very satisfying and unique type of practice that I will be adding more into my meditation routines, maybe with or without static stances or posture work.

Reference;
Pikörn, I. (2024, June 14). *The benefits of Tibetan singing bowls and how to use them*. Insight Timer Blog. https://insighttimer.com/blog/singing-bowls-meditation-benefits/

## Tummo, "inner fire" Meditation

Many of the posts here have discussed some of the mental or spiritual benefits of Tibetan Meditations. If appears as there is quite a bit of research on the physical benefits as well. Advanced methods of meditation, such as *Tummo*, may open up options that will help to better treat stress-related illnesses.

There are events reported where Tibetan monks have demonstrated some very high levels of meditation where they can perform seemingly miraculous feats of the human body. For instance, at a Buddhist monastery in Northern India, a group of monks were lightly dressed and unaffected by the temperature of their surroundings of 40 degrees Fahrenheit. They were then covered with ice-cold, wet sheets of fabric. An average person would be shivering uncontrollably to try to stay warm, however the monks remain unfazed. The wet sheets began to steam after about 1 hour, eventually becoming completely dry. The monks had used a yoga technique known as Tummo, which literally means 'inner fire'. This is an ancient meditation technique practiced by monks in Tibetan Buddhism. where a combination of breathing and visualization techniques are used to enter into a deep state of meditation. This method enabled them to significantly raise their body heat, as much as 17 degrees Fahrenheit in their fingers and toes.

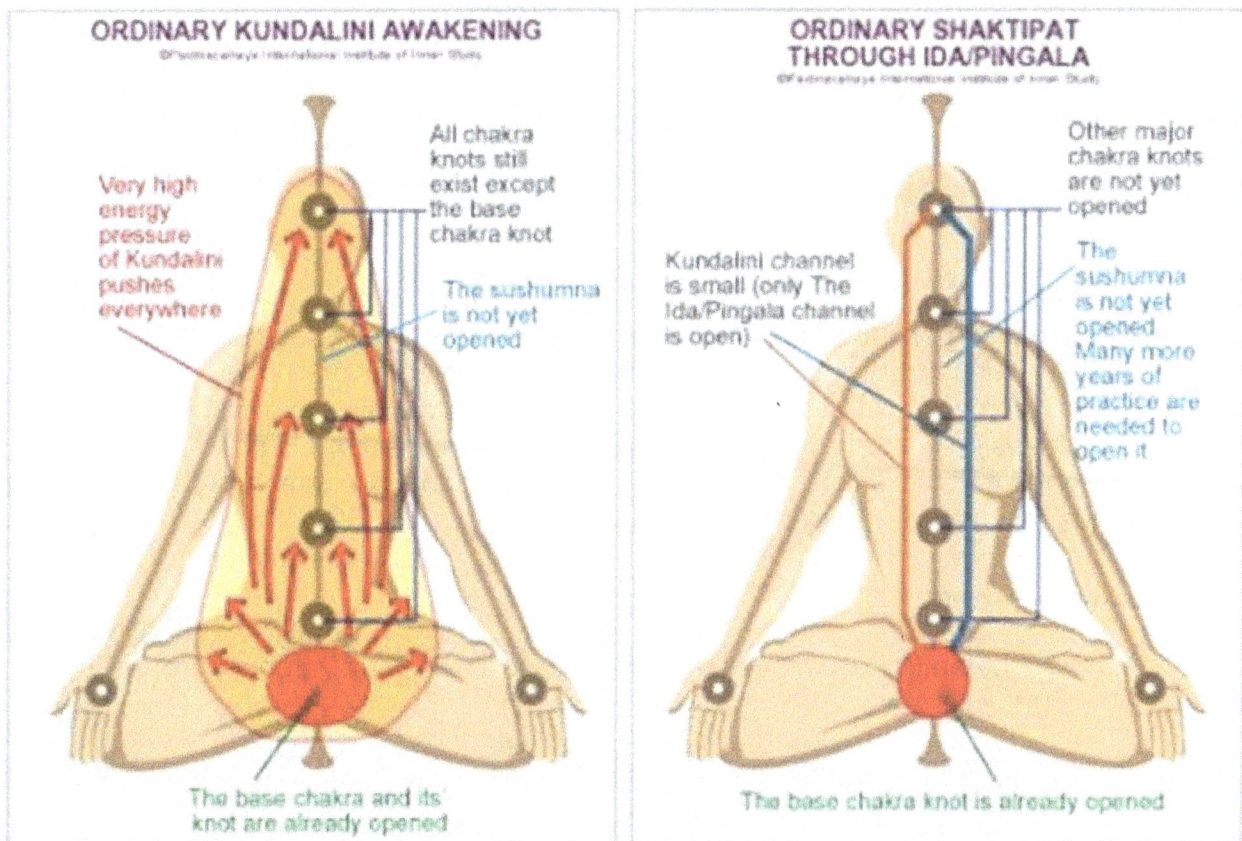

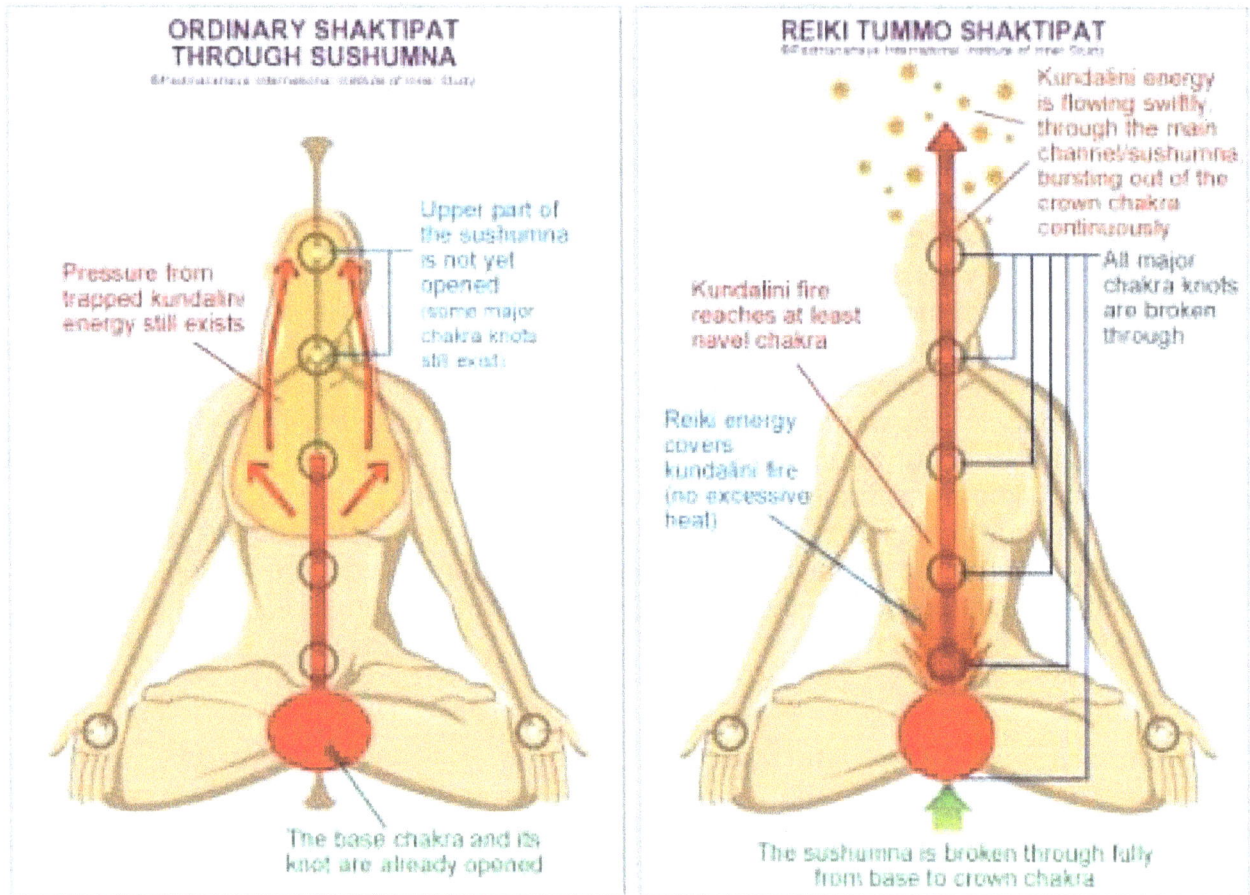

**ORDINARY SHAKTIPAT THROUGH SUSHUMNA**

Pressure from trapped kundalini energy still exists

Upper part of the sushumna is not yet opened (some major chakra knots still exist)

The base chakra and its knot are already opened

**REIKI TUMMO SHAKTIPAT**

Kundalini energy is flowing swiftly through the main channel/sushumna, bursting out of the crown chakra continuously

All major chakra knots are broken through

Kundalini fire reaches at least navel chakra

Reiki energy covers kundalini fire (no excessive heat)

The sushumna is broken through fully from base to crown chakra

http://35to65.com/meditation-sitting-snow-crazy-video-immune-function-tibetan-tummo-inner-heat-meditation/

Components of Tummo meditation that can lead to temperature increases are Vase breath and concentrative visualization. Vase breath is a particular breathing technique which causes thermogenesis, a process of heat production. Concentrative visualization is where the practitioner focuses on a mental image of flames along the spinal cord in order to prevent heat loss. Reports from scientists at Harvard University see this phenomenon as an amazing example of the mind's ability to influence the body.

References:

Explained: How Tibetan Monks Use Meditation to Raise Their Body Temperature (buzzworthy.com)

Tummo Meditation | Your Inner Fire and the Wim Hof Method

http://35to65.com/meditation-sitting-snow-crazy-video-immune-function-tibetan-tummo-inner-heat-meditation/

## What is Qi?

Qi is pronounced as "chee" and means "breath" in Chinese. Other definitions are vitality, energy, force, air, and vapor. Qi is the life energy that all living creatures require in order to exist. Different cultures call this energy Chi (English), Ki (from Japanese), Gi (Korean) or Prana (Indian). Qi is a type of energy in the human body and circulates within the blood, cells, and tissues throughout. "When qi moves, blood follows" is a root concept with Traditional Chinese Medicine (TCM). Qi flows in a specific pattern, at specific times from one organ to the next through meridians within the body. These meridians or channels might best be described as something similar to the electrical lines on a printed circuit board. There are 12 main meridians, with 2 for each organ (situated bilaterally from head to toe) for 12 organs. Zang Fu Zhi qi, is that which circulates through the organs. Jing Luo Zhi qi is that which circulates through the meridians.

Qi has mass the same way smoke or vapor has mass; both are transitional states of form. Qi (energy) is regarded as one of the 3 Treasures (San Jiao) or essential components of life, with essence (Jing) and spirit (Shen) being the other two. When energy, essence and spirit are in harmony with one another, the person finds themselves alert, healthy, and vibrant. Or the opposite if their treasures are in imbalance. If this harmonious flow is disrupted, illness occurs.

• Physically *(jing):* energetically manifesting as the body's cells and tissues into form, bone marrow, blood and bodily fluids.

• Energetically *(qi):* as resonant vibration, heat, sound, light and electromagnetic fields.

• Spiritually *(shen):* energetically manifesting through subtle vibrations which extend through space or Wu Ji.

The following graphic shows how qi can be conceptualized into the Chinese ideogram of rice cooking atop a heat source and producing the wisps of vapor (energy) that we see rising above the cooking rice.

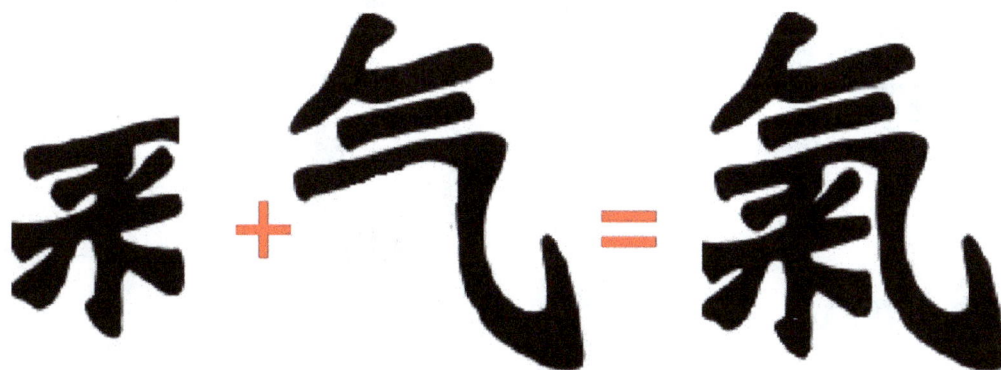

米 + 气 = 氣

| grain of rice | wisp of steam | qi |

The amount of qi in one's body and the quality of it determines whether an individual is generally healthy or prone to illness. There is a finite amount in our bodies and is gradually exhausted due to age and possible abuses. When it decreases so does the lifespan of the individual.

A proper balance of nutrition, exercise and a healthy lifestyle directly affects the quality and abundance of qi. Emotions and their balance or lack thereof affect the quality of an individual's qi. The emotions of joy, anger, sadness, grief and fear affect our qi within specific organs.

# *qi* = life force

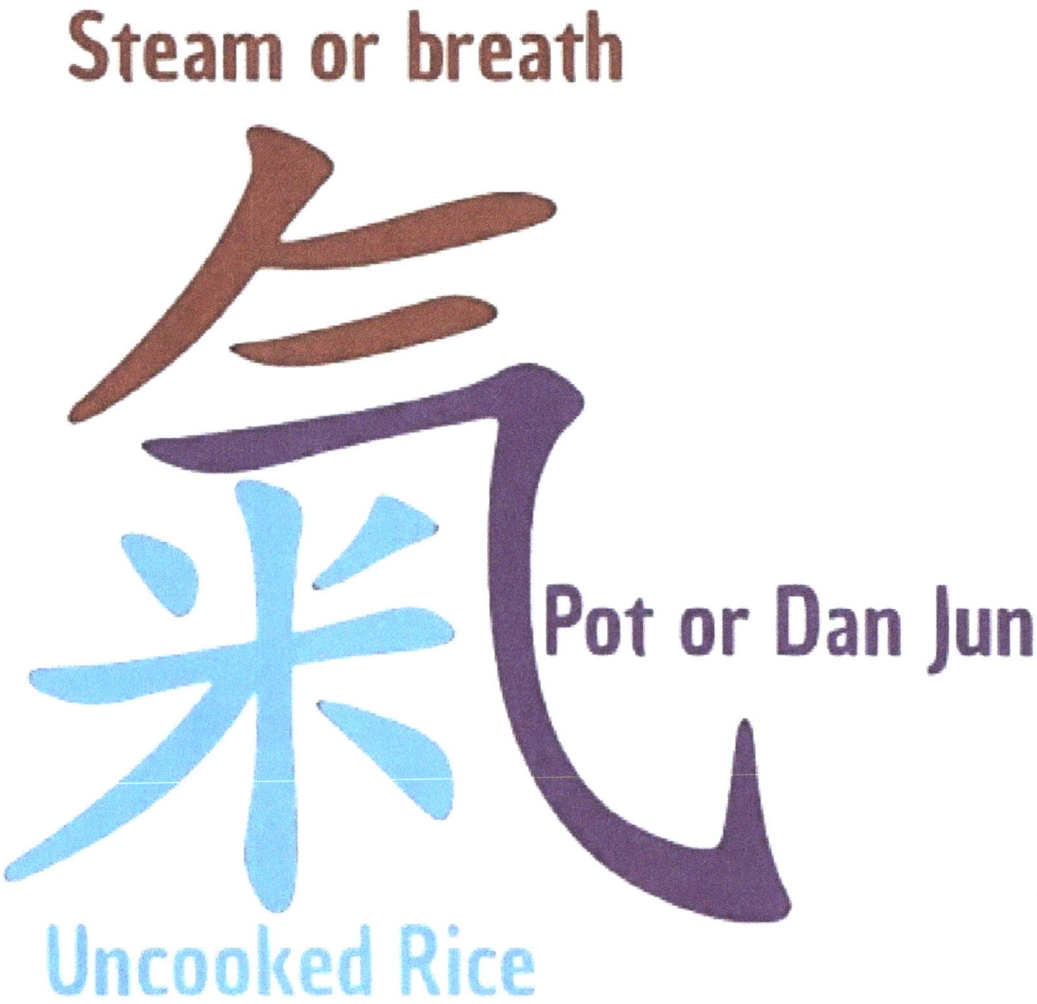

**Steam or breath**

**Pot or Dan Jun**

**Uncooked Rice**

**Qi, Chi** or **Gi** means air, energy or breath in Chinese and Korean. Gong or Kung means work. Qigong therefore translates to energy or breath work. This "work" or exercises are also referred to as Chi Kung and Gi Gong.

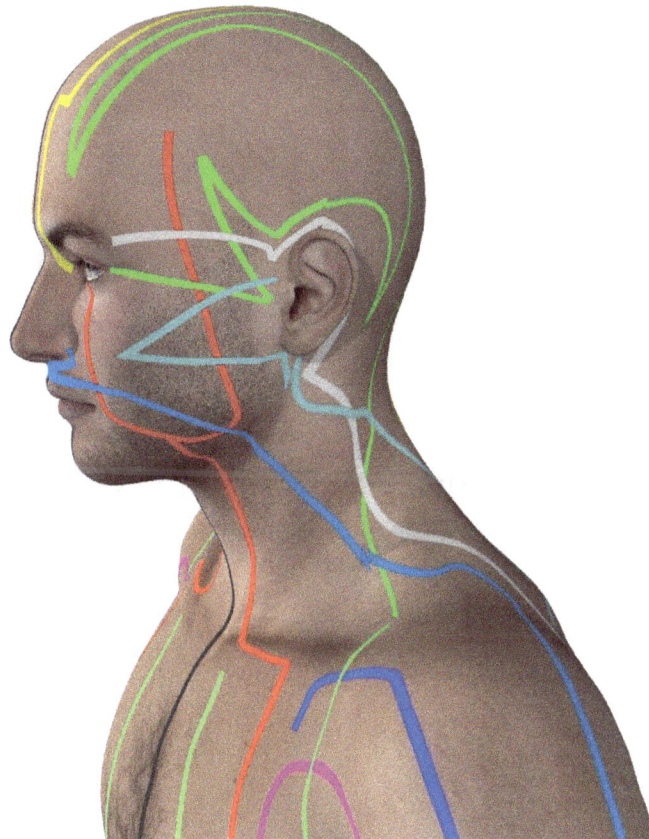

The human body is made up of bones, muscles, and organs amongst other components. Veins, arteries and capillaries carry blood and nutrients throughout to all of the systems and components. Additionally, 12 major energy medians carry the body's energy. "life force" also known as "qi". Ones qi is stored in the lower Dan Tien. Daily emotional imbalances accumulate tension and stress gradually affecting all of the body's systems. Each discomfort, nuisance, irritation or grudge continues to tighten and squeeze the flow of the life force. This is where "dis-ease" claims its foothold.

Qigong breathing exercises can adjust the brainwaves to the Alpha state where the mind is relaxed and the body chemistry changes and promotes natural healing. Relaxing of the deep skeletal muscles, working outward. Release of tension accumulated within the muscles, organs and nerves. Whereas conventional physical exercise can deplete energy, Qigong helps to replenish your natural energy.

Similar to a sponge, the body absorbs positive as well as negative energy . Each emotion effects an internal organ. Qi Gong helps to balance the emotions:

Liver - anger, depression
Heart - excess of joy
Spleen - worry
Lung - grief
Kidney - fear

Grief Fear
Excess of Joy
Anger Worry

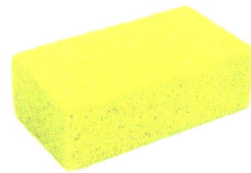

Healthy Sponge     Compressed Sponge

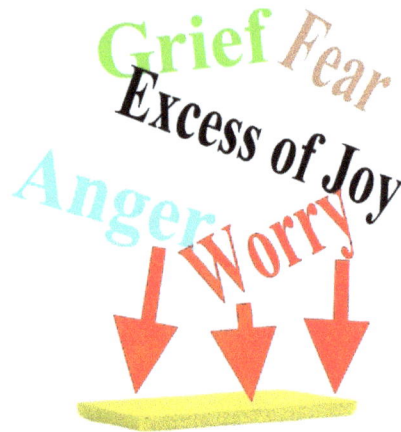

Our emotional state directly influences how we breathe. The emotions reveal themselves in the breathing patterns:

**Anger, fear, anxiety** - shallow breaths

**Grief** - spasmodic breathing

**Guilt** - restricted breathing

**Boredom** - shallow, lifeless breathing

**Sadness/depression** - under breathing

Furthermore:

**Dwelling in the past** - can produce any of the above breathing patterns

**Worrying about the future** - can produce any of the above breathing patterns

**Present in the moment** - The goal here is clarity and self-awareness to slow and regulate the breath

**Basic Qigong exercise:**

1) Stand, sit or lay in a position as shown to the right.

2) Try to align the body as shown in figure to the right, while remaining relaxed.

3) Inhale and exhale through the nose as the tongue gently touches the roof of the mouth behind the teeth.

4) Relax the forehead, eyebrows, eyelids, eyes, cheeks, lips and the jaw. close the mouth but don't clench your teeth.

5) Close the eyes to take away the distractions of what your eyes see.

6) Try to picture your body in your thought as you begin a scan from the top of your head working downward towards the toes.

7) As you think of the different parts of the body, try to imagine the deep skeletal muscles releasing from the bones as if they were melting or dissolving away.

8) Continue to become more self-aware of where you are holding tension within the body. As you exhale, try to release any tension in those areas by "dissolving" it away.

9) Follow your breath from the diaphragm as you fill the lungs from bottom to top.

10) Let the stomach muscles pull inward as exhaling and bringing your thought back downward to just below the navel to the "Lower Dan Tien".

11) Continue this process as long or little as you choose, mindful that longer periods of time don't necessarily reflect increased benefits if not performed correctly. However, most benefits are arrived at over a period of time with consistent practice.

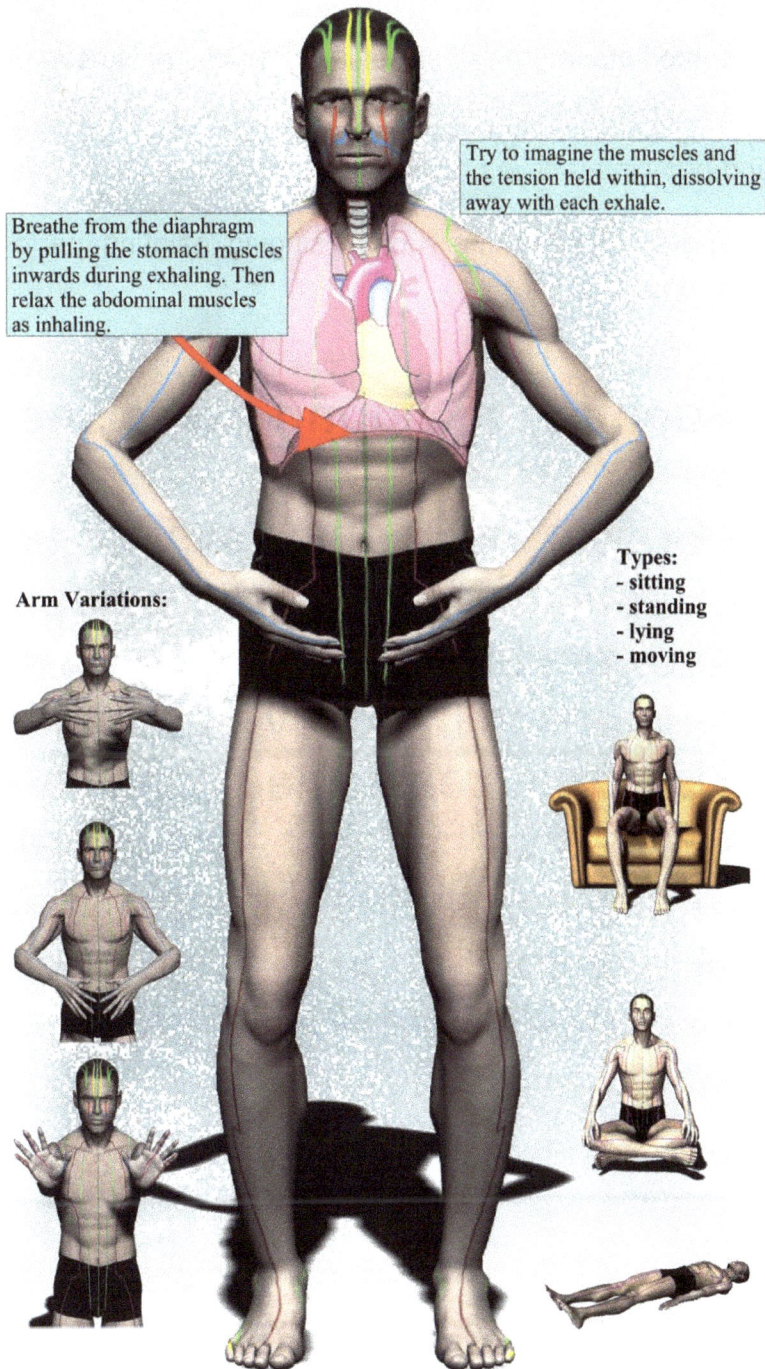

© Copyright 2018 - CAD Graphics, Inc.

Breathe from the diaphragm by pulling the stomach muscles inwards during exhaling. Then relax the abdominal muscles as inhaling.

Try to imagine the muscles and the tension held within, dissolving away with each exhale.

**Arm Variations:**

**Types:**
- sitting
- standing
- lying
- moving

Becoming present in the moment can happen in various ways such as:

1) Immediate trauma - Fear of injury or loss of life can put one into the moment quickly.

2) Practice of mindful exercises such as meditation, yoga, tai chi, qigong and other similar mind and body interactive practices.

3) Engaging in activities such as singing, painting, performing music, dancing, etc.

**Benefits of Qigong exercises:**

- Boosts the immune system
- Reduces stress, anxiety, depression, mood swings
- Lowers blood pressure
- Increases the body's natural healing process
- Lungs increase their capacity
- Promotes better respiration and circulation
- Enhanced self-awareness
- Helps to change the body's chemistry for the better

------------

**The 8 Extraordinary Energy Meridians or Vessels**

## Control What You Can - YOU

Similar to a sponge, the mind and body absorb positive as will as negative energy. Each emotion affects an internal organ. Exercises such as meditation, yoga, tai chi and others can help to balance our emotions.

Liver - anger, depression
Heart - excess of joy
Spleen - worry
Lung - grief
Kidney - fear

*Grief Fear*
*Excess of Joy*
*Anger*
*Worry*

Healthy Sponge          Compressed Sponge

© Copyright 2022 - CAD Graphics, Inc. www.MindandBodyExercises.com

Life's Challenges Pressing Inwards
Work
Internal Strife
Family
Your Consciousness
Culture
School     Society     Friends

You Pressing Stresses Outwards

You Realizing That You Control You

**NO CONTROL**
Feeling like others control your thoughts, actions and life

**SELF-CONTROL**
Choosing to do what is right, in spite of your personal gain or loss

By strengthening the physical body through exercise – specific exercises such as yoga, tai chi, qigong, and others, are methods to develop self-disciple. By practicing self-induced strategic trauma (training) one can dramatically strengthen their nervous system and in turn develop mental stress to better deal with the stress of daily trials and tribulations. By manifesting our own internal pressure (mind and body training), it is much easier to manage external pressure (stress) that constantly pushes into our personal space.

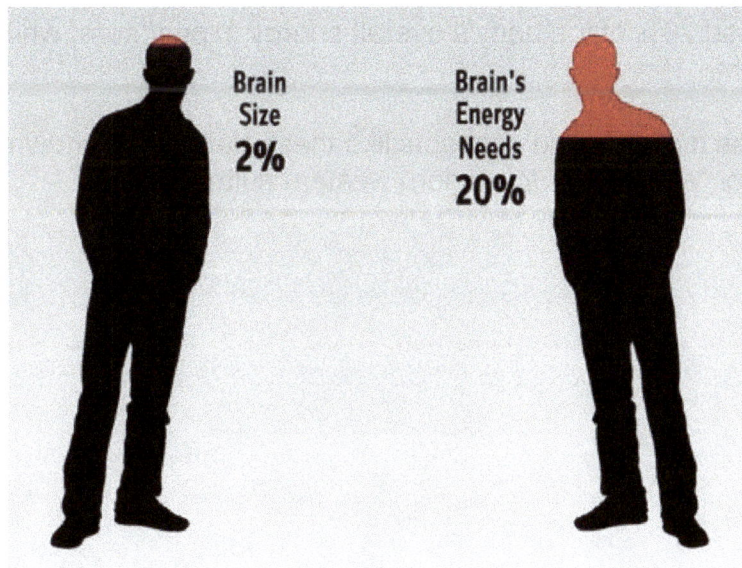

Brain Size 2%

Brain's Energy Needs 20%

# The Eight Extraordinary Meridians (energetic structure)

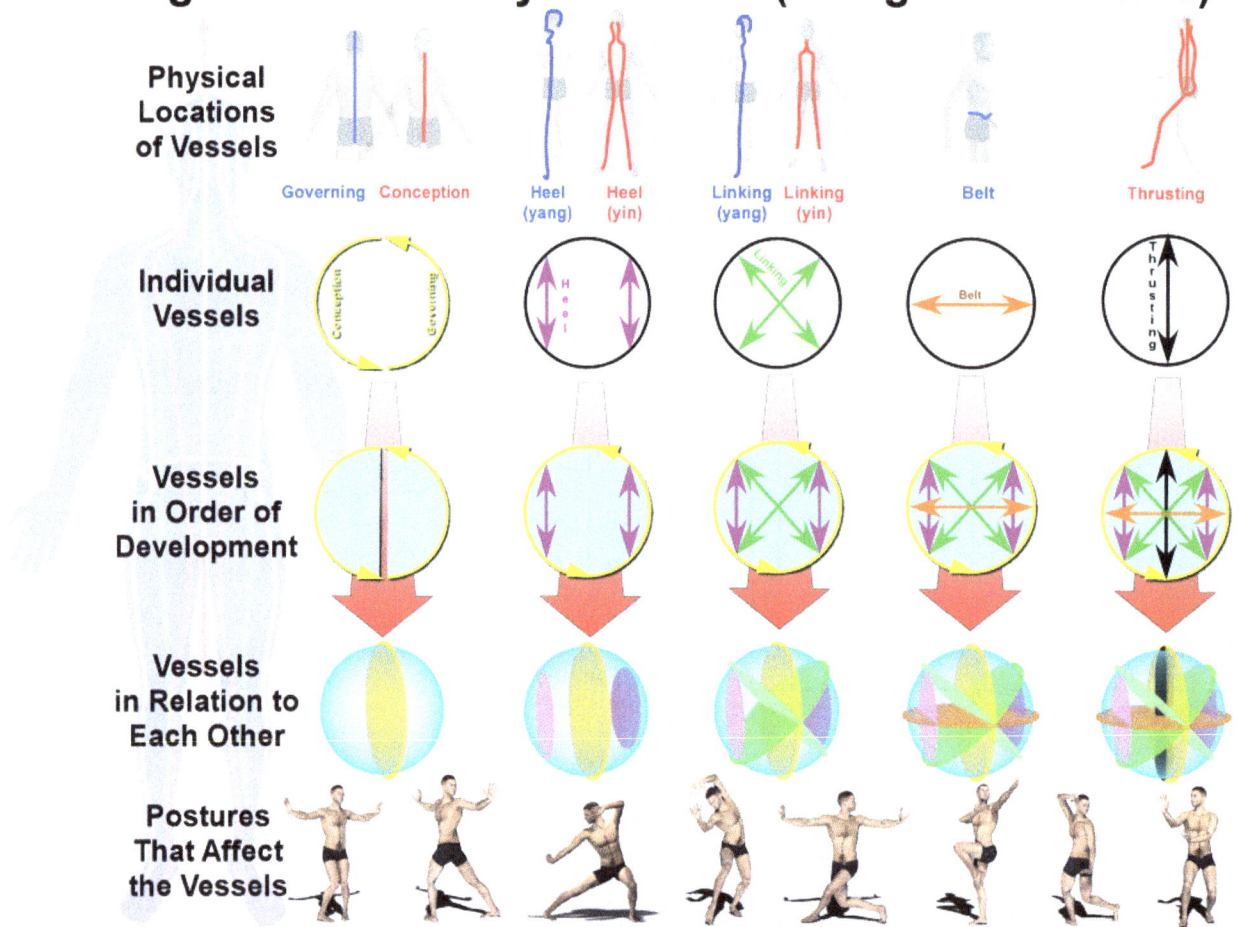

| | Governing | Conception | Heel (yang) | Heel (yin) | Linking (yang) | Linking (yin) | Belt | Thrusting |
|---|---|---|---|---|---|---|---|---|
| Physical Locations of Vessels | | | | | | | | |
| Individual Vessels | | | | | | | | |
| Vessels in Order of Development | | | | | | | | |
| Vessels in Relation to Each Other | | | | | | | | |
| Postures That Affect the Vessels | | | | | | | | |

www.MindAndBodyExercises.com

© Copyright 2020 - CAD Graphics, Inc.

Managing one's physical body, thoughts and emotions all burn a tremendous amount of energy. The brain used 20% of the body's overall energy expenditure, while only comprising 2% of our body weight.

Exercise and wellness methods and concepts like these have been known for centuries but are considered new or "alternative" to modern western culture.

# Where Energy is used in the Body?

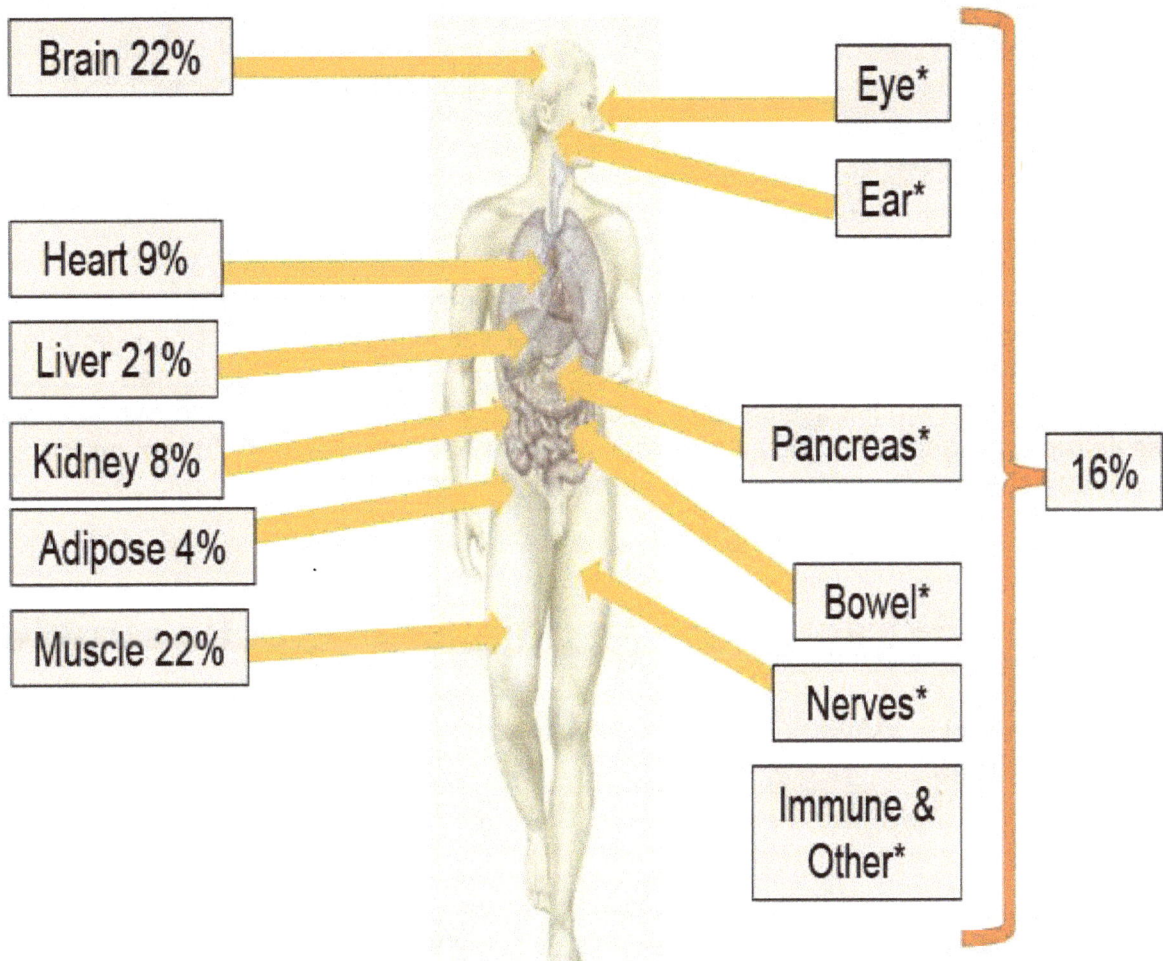

| | | |
|---|---|---|
| Brain 22% | Eye* | |
| | Ear* | |
| Heart 9% | | |
| Liver 21% | | |
| Kidney 8% | Pancreas* | 16% |
| Adipose 4% | | |
| Muscle 22% | Bowel* | |
| | Nerves* | |
| | Immune & Other* | |

Fatigue and Vitality – Saskatoon Wellness Centre (saskwellness.com)

Building stronger muscles can lead to building stronger joints and bones. Additionally, by holding static postures, positions or exercises the nervous system is strengthened. Specific joint alignments engage the nervous system to endure more pain, stress and discomfort. Standing perfectly for 1 minute can be challenging; 5 minutes of not moving might be considered self-torture for some. And that is just standing and not even trying to hold a difficult posture. Think of tempering steel in fire to strengthen the metal.

# The Eight Extraordinary Meridians (energetic structure)

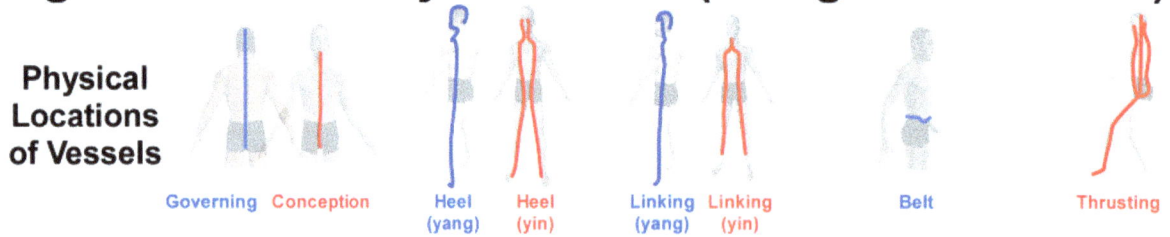

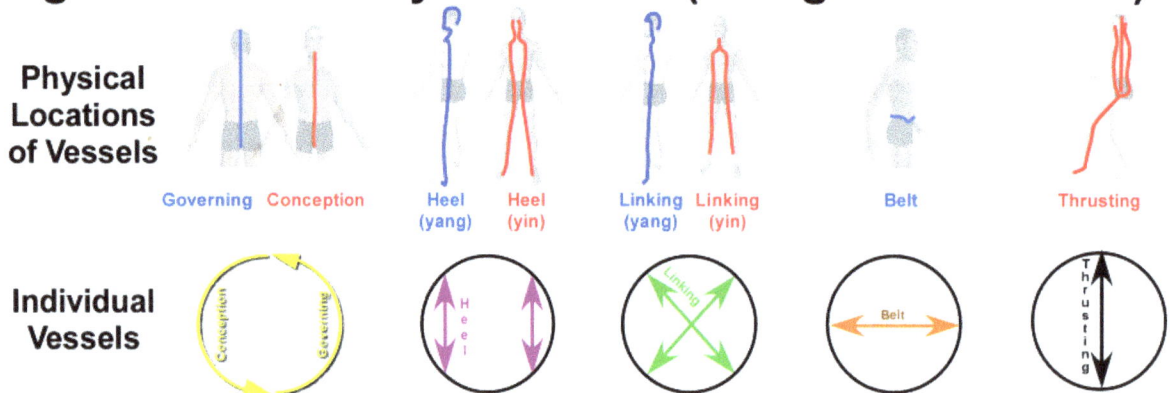

**Physical Locations of Vessels**

Governing  Conception  Heel (yang)  Heel (yin)  Linking (yang)  Linking (yin)  Belt  Thrusting

When engaging in the muscles, tendons, bones and fascia, the 12 regular energy meridians are engaged plus the 8 extraordinary meridians (or vessels) are opened and filled as reservoirs to adjust the ebb and flow of energy throughout the body and thereby strengthening the immune system among other bodily functions. These meridians and vessels run throughout the body in a spider web-like pattern from head to toe, on the surface as well as deep into the internals of the human body.

# The Eight Extraordinary Meridians (energetic structure)

**Physical Locations of Vessels**

Governing  Conception  Heel (yang)  Heel (yin)  Linking (yang)  Linking (yin)  Belt  Thrusting

**Individual Vessels**

Often times people will ask me, "where did you learn this?" Well…almost 40 years ago I began studying Korean kung fu, then Traditional Chinese Medicine, medical qigong, fitness, wellness and anatomy. It didn't happen overnight or from a weekend seminar. It took me decades of learning, studying and teaching from and with high level masters and teachers. And I'm not done learning yet, are you?

# The Eight Extraordinary Meridians (energetic structure)

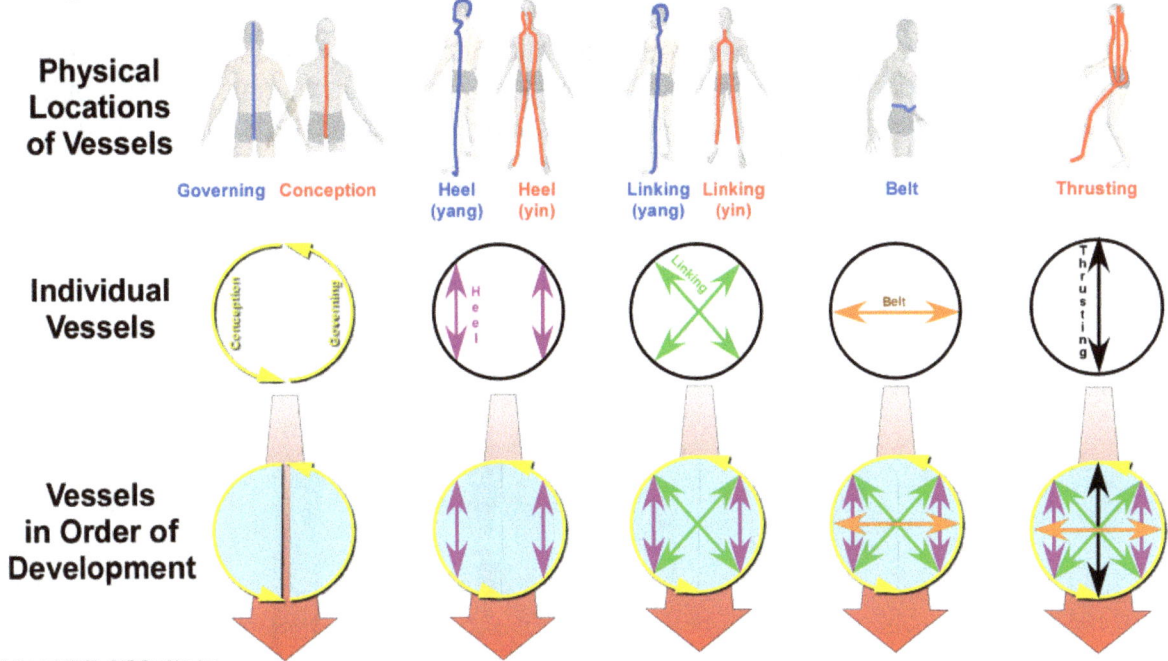

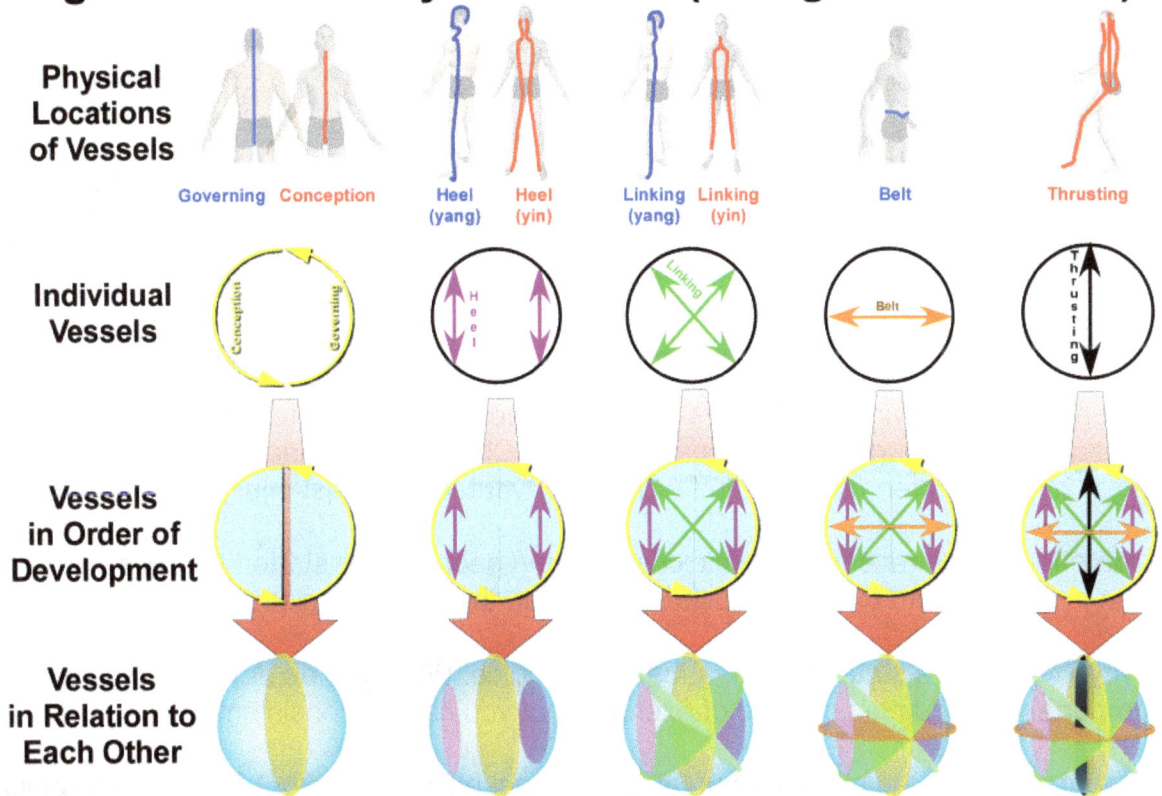

**Physical Locations of Vessels**

Governing　Conception　Heel (yang)　Heel (yin)　Linking (yang)　Linking (yin)　Belt　Thrusting

**Individual Vessels**

**Vessels in Order of Development**

© Copyright 2020 - CAD Graphics, Inc.

# The Eight Extraordinary Meridians (energetic structure)

**Physical Locations of Vessels**

Governing　Conception　Heel (yang)　Heel (yin)　Linking (yang)　Linking (yin)　Belt　Thrusting

**Individual Vessels**

**Vessels in Order of Development**

**Vessels in Relation to Each Other**

© Copyright 2020 - CAD Graphics, Inc.

## Stretching of the Fascial Trains

Fascia is a band or layer of connective tissue, mostly comprised of collagen, which lies beneath the skin and attaches, stabilizes, engages, and separates muscles and other internal organs. These layers are integrated and interconnected within bands that runs from the bottom of the feet to top of the head.

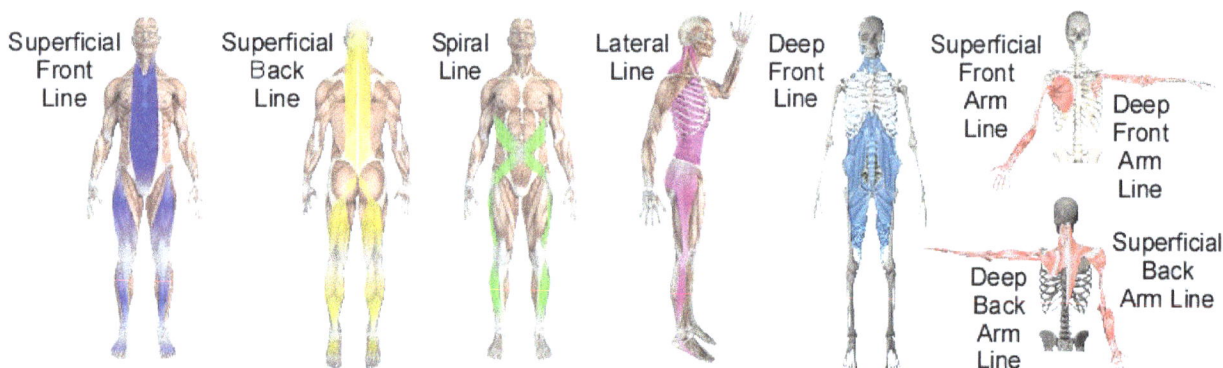

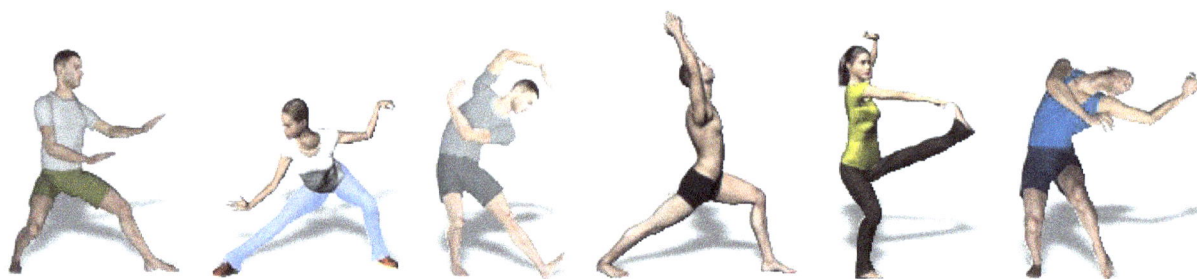

Superficial Front Line
Superficial Back Line
Spiral Line
Lateral Line
Deep Front Line
Superficial Front Arm Line
Deep Front Arm Line
Deep Back Arm Line
Superficial Back Arm Line

There are many individual exercises and techniques that can stretch and release tension of the fascia trains throughout the human body. Tai Chi, Qigong, Yoga and Pilates are methods of stretching and strengthening the fascia as preventative or post-injury low impact exercises.

A side effect of the recent pandemic crisis - some people have started to realize that good health is not all about the location, the equipment, the gear, the clothes, the look.

Staying healthy is a state of mind, a matter of choice. What you do or where you do it is not as important as finding a method of exercise that you can do consistently.

The goal here is not to get a strenuous high-impact physical workout, but rather to build strength in all of the muscles, joints, bones, fascia and all other components of the human body. These exercises can be practiced aerobically (moving) to engage the circulatory system or anaerobically (holding each posture) with deep and deliberate breathing to engage the parasympathetic nervous system.

As we all continue to age, the focus should change somewhat from the cosmetic attraction of a lean and toned physique to that of structurally sound and healthy internal systems. Most people don't ail from weak biceps or un-toned stomach and chest muscles. It is the health underneath that is most important.

These exercises have passed the test of time. Yoga/qigong (origins in 3300-1500 BCE), Asian Martial Arts (origins of 4-5 century AD), Tai Chi (origins in 12th century AD).

These practices have endured because they produce results for those that take them seriously.

https://youtu.be/7sxXXQuDX5c?si=SLfYAbJbT8JT7KAi

Thai massage seems to work heavily with the physical concept of myofascial release, that can be seen in Rolfing and other massage methods that have evolved over the last few centuries. However, Thai massage appears to have originated thousands of years ago. Also, I see Thai massage as a more mutually engaging type of practice where both the patient and practitioner seem to both be engaged in the goal of better health and well-being for both.

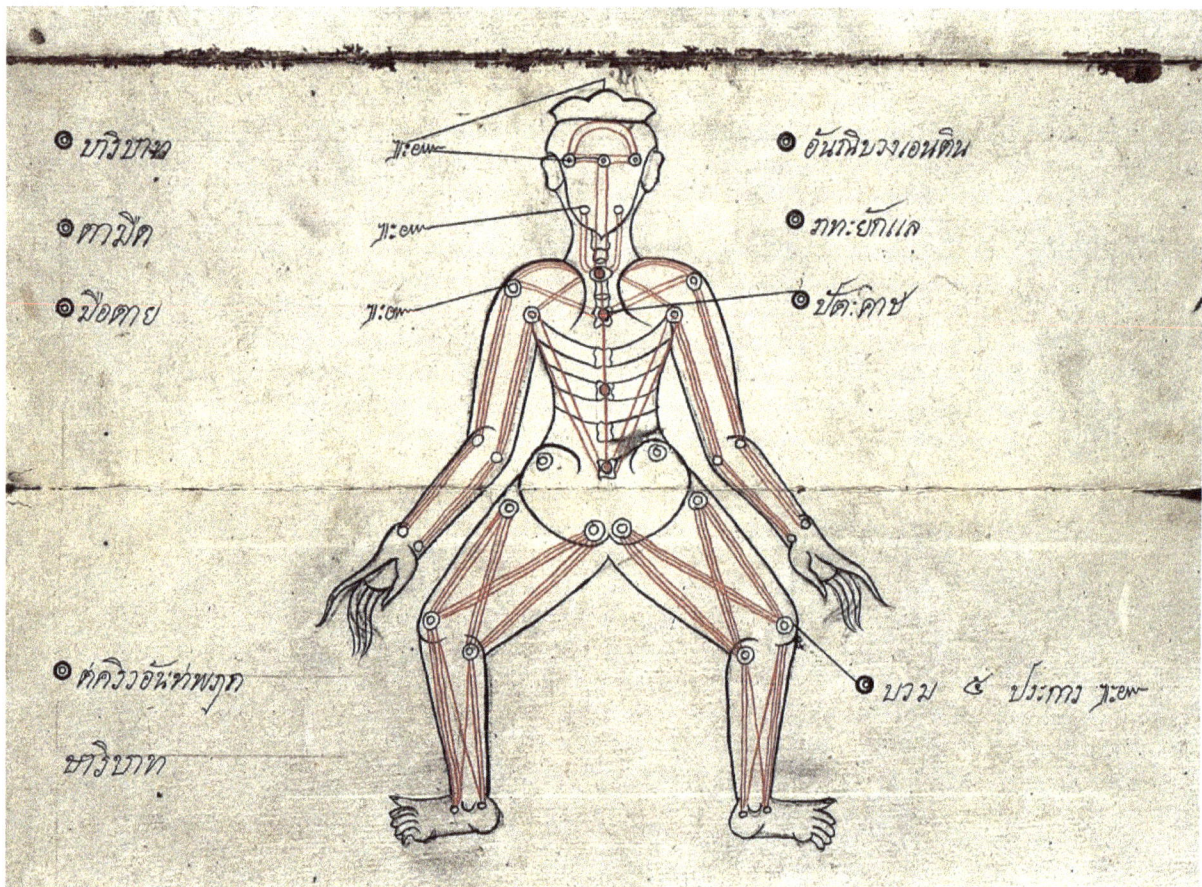

L0027324 Siamese Manuscript, Pressure Massage Manual. Credit: Wellcome Library, London. Wellcome Images images@wellcome.ac.uk http://wellcomeimages.org A guide to pressure points for use in 'Thai Yoga Massage'. Diagram: human figure showing pressure points. circa 1850 Published: - Copyrighted work available under Creative Commons Attribution only licence CC BY 4.0 http://creativecommons.org/licenses/by/4.0/

Thai massage has deep roots in its origins in Buddhism and yoga. Very similar to TCM concepts of energy flow throughout the body by way of the meridians or *sens*. The yoga concepts of chakras do align with the Chinese meridian system of TCM. Direct pressure on key points (acupoints) are preferred over kneading of the skin, fascia and muscles. Thai massage is composed of foundation concepts of meditation, postures or stances, rhythmic rocking, and other touch/pressure techniques. Meditation appears to be a very strong component, where the practitioner is actively involved in the present moment. By being engaged with the patient on the 3 levels of mind, body and spirit they are able to help the patient through applying loving kindness or *"metta"* to their patient.

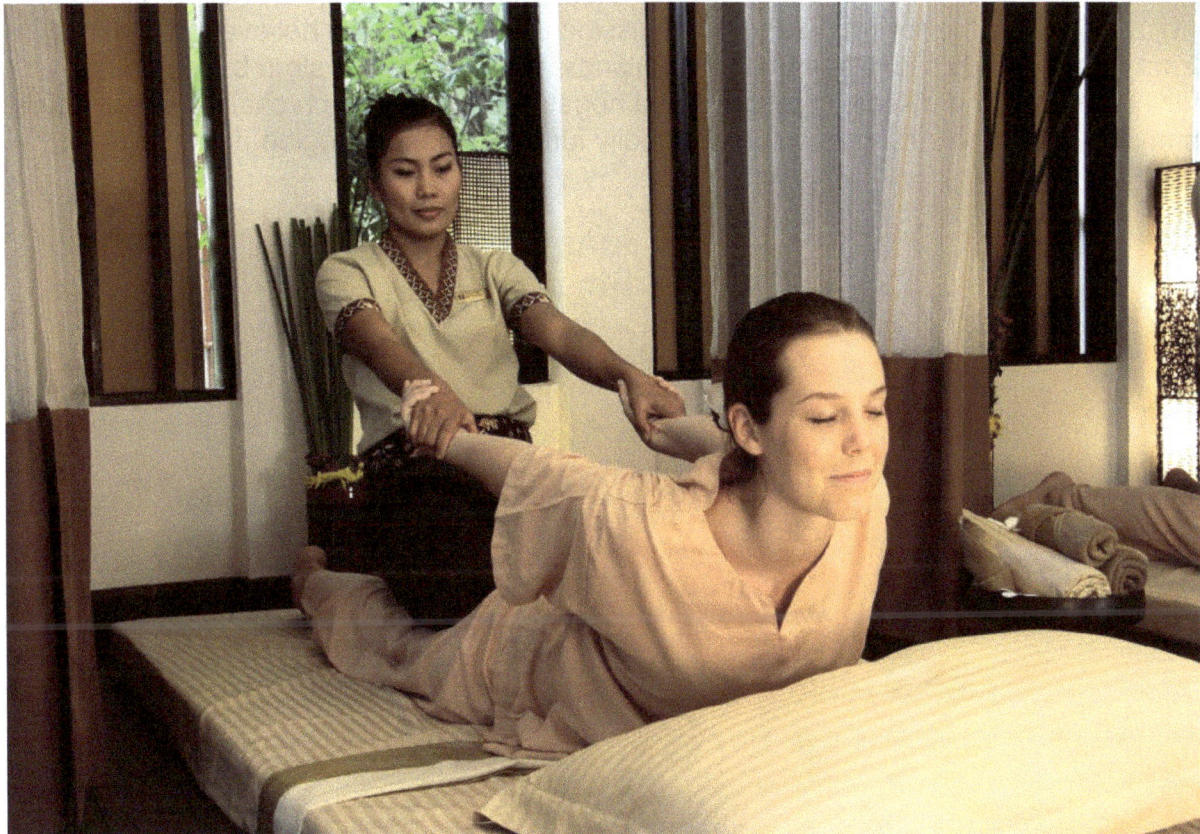

Thai massage has deep roots in its origins in yoga from Jivaka Kumar Bhaccha developing it over 2500 years ago. This method of healthcare does appear to me to embody the concept of balancing the mind, body and spirit where if one aspect is out of harmony with the others, disease, illness and suffering will manifest. As with any of these time proven practices that have been passed on for thousands of years, there must be something here regardless of Western allopathic Medicine's resistance to recognizing the benefits of these mind, body and spiritual methods of healthcare and well-being.

It is my understanding from many of the modern Western massage practitioners that I have visited that they often feel exhausted not just after the individual sessions but accumulatively over the time of their career. I found this more prevalent when the massage therapists themselves did not practice taking care of themselves to replenish the energy that they put out during the massage treatments. Those that I have met that cared to share told me that it was essential for them to practice something like yoga, tai chi, qigong, meditation as well as good nutrition to stay balanced, as far as energy conservation goes. I have learned that we cannot give out freely, which we do not already have an abundance of without some level of detriment to all involved.

Chakra is a Sanskrit word that means "wheel." Chakras and Dimensions are the same thing. Sometimes they will be referred to as the "Seven *Dantians*." Coming from traditional Indian medicine, there exist 7 energy centers within the human body. These points are considered the focal points for the reception and transmission of energy. Some believe the chakras interact with the body's ductless endocrine glands and lymphatic system by feeding in positive energies and disposing of unwanted negative energies. Each chakra in your spinal column is believed to influence our direct bodily functions near its region of the spine.

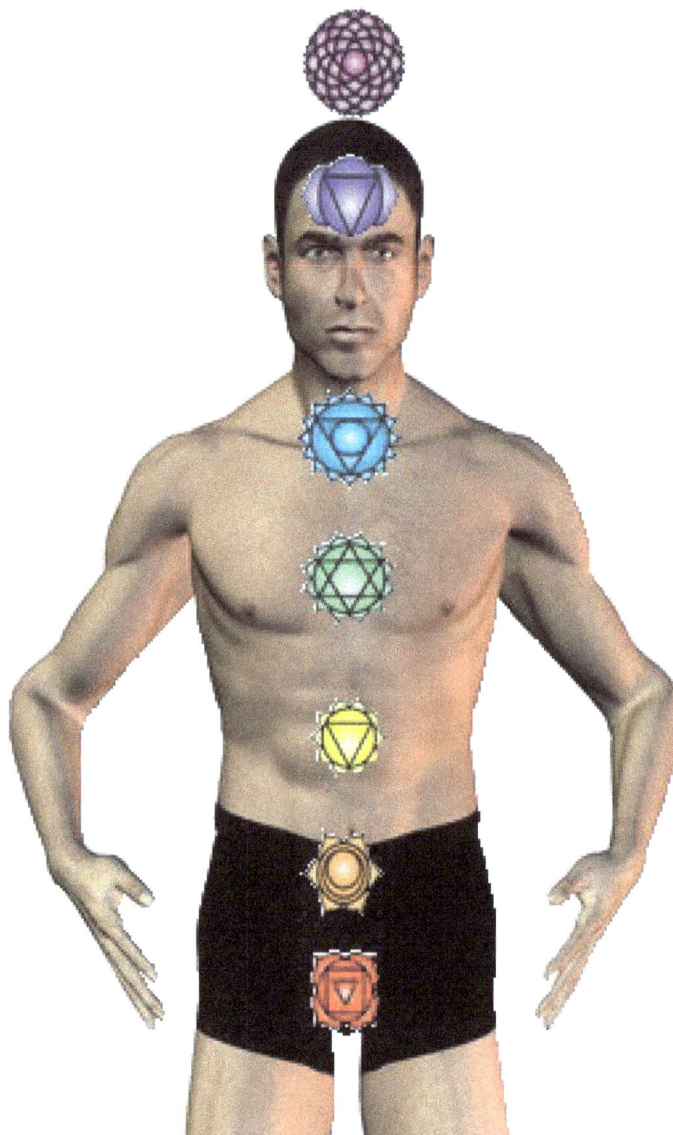

Chakras are energy systems associated with different parts of the body that relay information in the form of energy. It is believed that a chakra is a wheel of energy that spins around its own axis and can spin fast or slowly. These chakras are like spirals of energy, each one relating to the others. A chakra will spin in relation to the energy level of your system, thus understanding your chakras and keeping them in balance can help with all kinds of health and emotional problems.

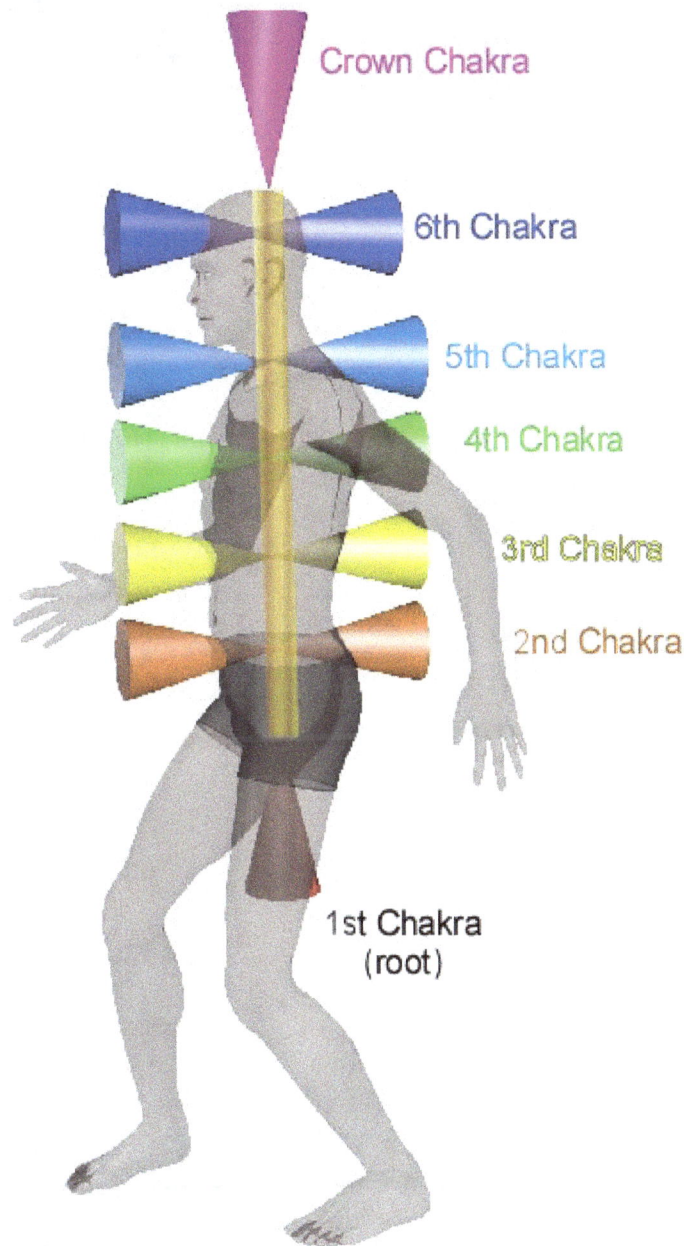

Crown Chakra

6th Chakra

5th Chakra

4th Chakra

3rd Chakra

2nd Chakra

1st Chakra
(root)

**You can think of chakras as invisible, rechargeable batteries.**
Imagine a vertical power current like a fluorescent tube that runs up and down the spine, from the top of the head to the base of the spine. Think of this as your main source of energy. The seven major chakras are in the center of the body and are aligned with this vertical "power line."

They regulate the flow of energy throughout the electrical network (Meridians) that runs through the physical body. The body's electrical system resembles the wiring in a house. It allows electrical current to be sent to every part and is ready for use when needed.

# The 12 Primary Energy Meridians

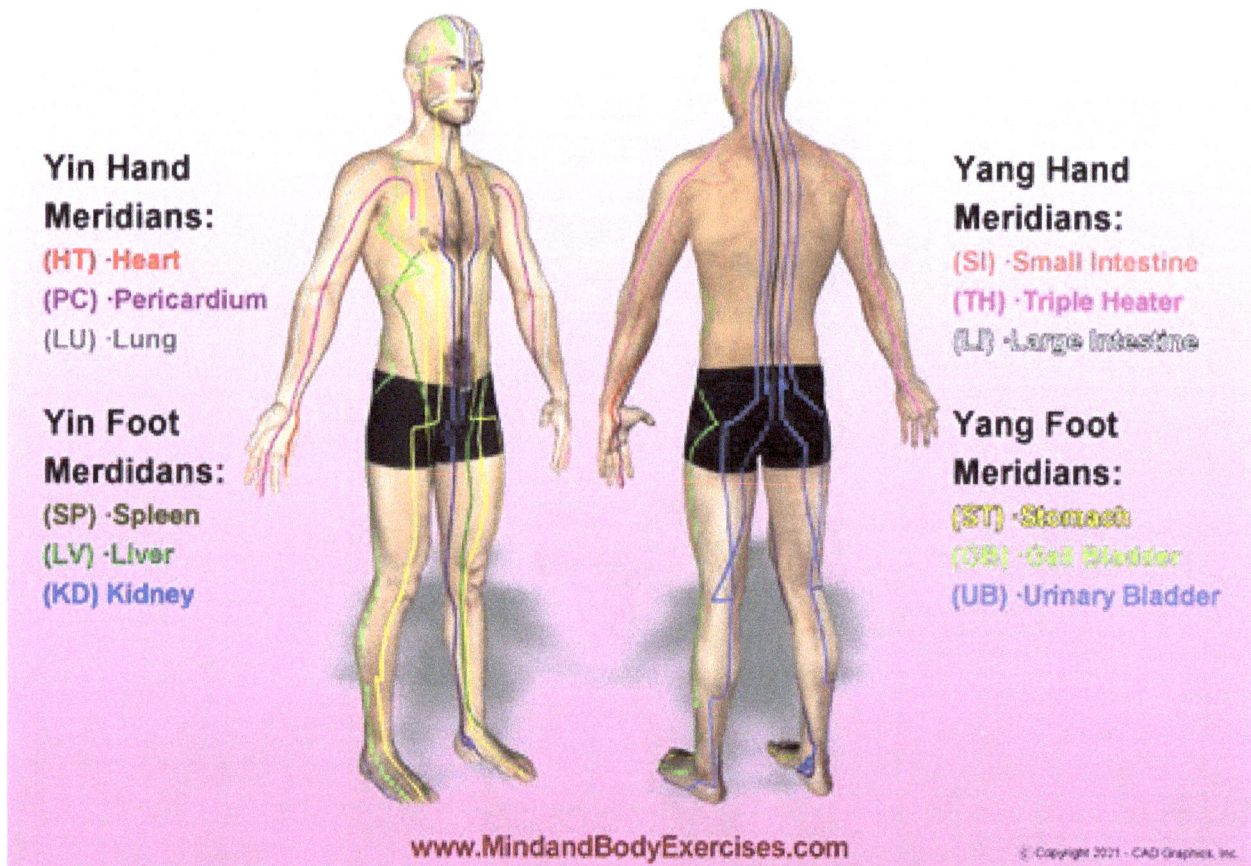

**Yin Hand Meridians:**
(HT) ·Heart
(PC) ·Pericardium
(LU) ·Lung

**Yin Foot Meridians:**
(SP) ·Spleen
(LV) ·Liver
(KD) Kidney

**Yang Hand Meridians:**
(SI) ·Small Intestine
(TH) ·Triple Heater
(LI) ·Large Intestine

**Yang Foot Meridians:**
(ST) ·Stomach
(GB) ·Gall Bladder
(UB) ·Urinary Bladder

www.MindandBodyExercises.com

© Copyright 2021 - CAD Graphics, Inc.

Sometimes chakras become blocked because of stress, emotional or physical problems. If the body's "energy system" cannot flow freely it is likely that problems will occur. The consequence of irregular energy flow may result in physical illness and discomfort or a sense of being mentally and emotionally out of balance. Blocked energy in our Seven Chakras can often lead to illness so it's important to understand what each Chakra represents and what we can do to keep this energy flowing freely.

| Start with the root and crown energy centers | Then divide the body into 3 sections | Then split each of the 3 sections in half. The connecting energy points create the 7 Chakras or dimensions |
|---|---|---|

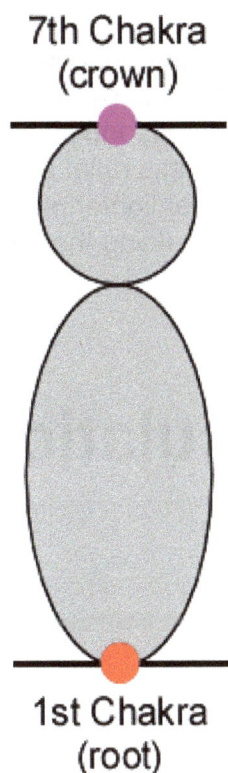

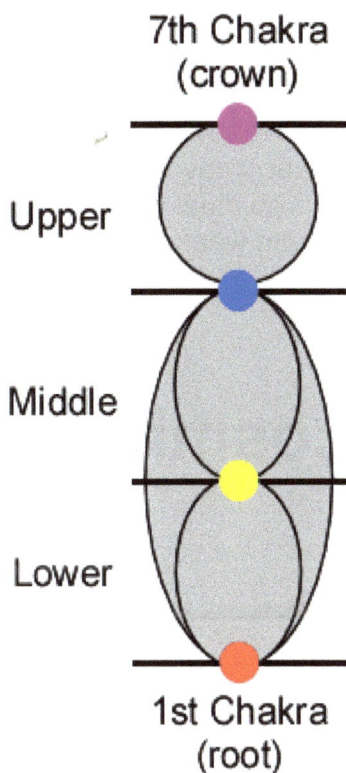

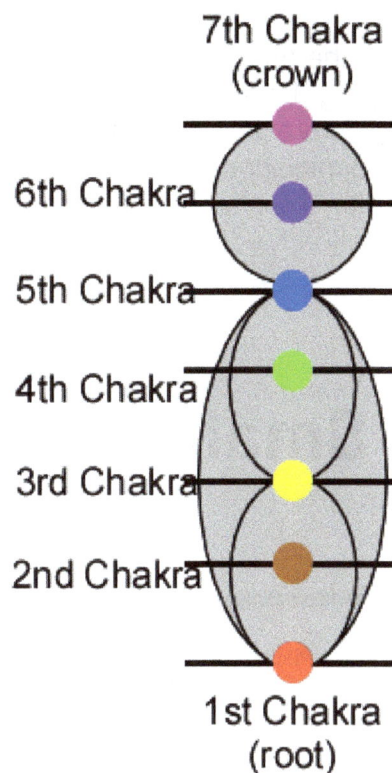

**7th Chakra (crown)**

**Upper**

**Middle**

**Lower**

6th Chakra

5th Chakra

4th Chakra

3rd Chakra

2nd Chakra

**1st Chakra (root)**

The universe contains an infinite number of dimensions of existence. There are seven that are part of the "human experience." There are infinite dimensions above our "7th Dimension" and infinite dimensions below our "1st Dimension." We can concern ourselves with seven, however it is important to understand that just as the universe keeps expanding, so do the dimensions. You could even say that there are "infinity + 1" dimensions. That statement points to the ever-expanding universe.

**Heaven and Earth**
Man, literally stands in between heaven and earth. Heaven begins at your crown chakra – 1/infinity of an inch above your *bahui* point. Earth begins at the bottom of your foot (K1). If we look at the "energetic body" we just look at the head, midsection and torso. In other words, everything but the arms and legs.

The Small Circulation, Small Circle, or the Microcosmic Orbit, is the practice of circulating one's internal energy (Qi or chi), within the human body. The illustration below represents the awareness of energy flow throughout the Governing and Conception meridians, in this case, the fire path. These meridians are located on the center line of the body and in turn govern and regulate the other meridians. This practice has been considered to be the foundation of Internal Qigong. It was a fundamental step on the path of meditation training in ancient times. Over time, this practice has gradually been lost from many meditation traditions, and its importance diminished. Though meditation is popular today for relaxation, stress relief and general health, the ultimate goal for some people is spiritual awareness and enlightenment. Small Circulation Meditation transforms the body from weak to strong while training the mind to be calm and focused.

# The Small or Microcosmic Circulation

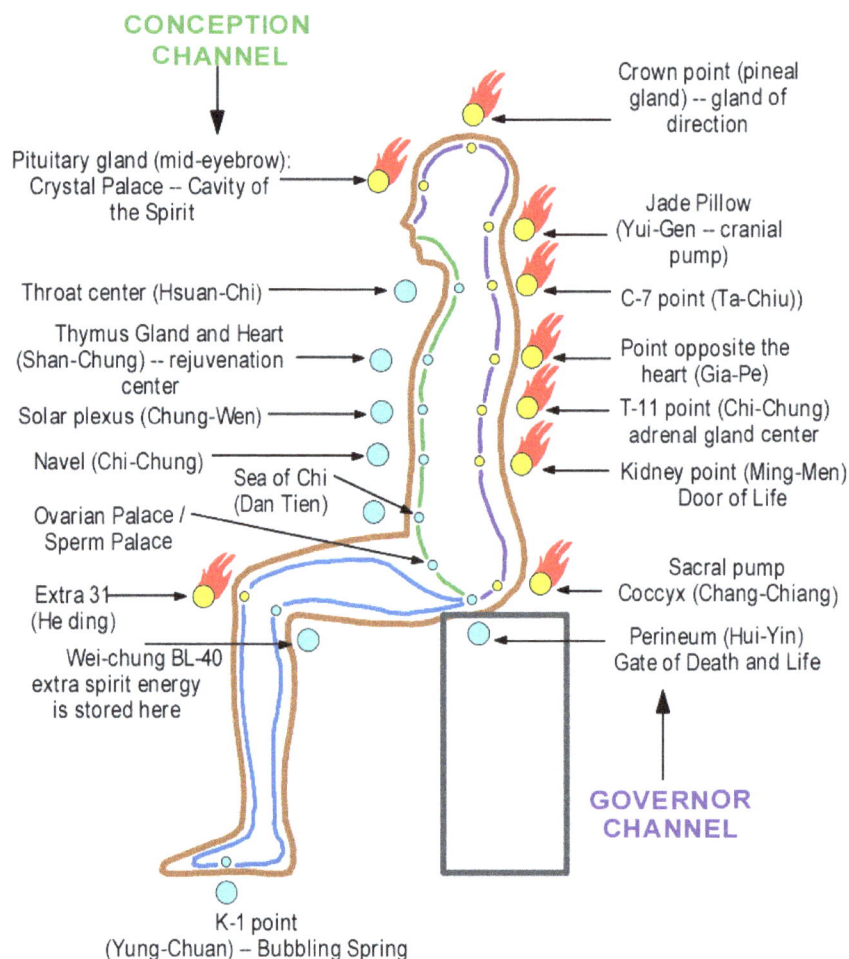

CONCEPTION CHANNEL

Crown point (pineal gland) -- gland of direction

Pituitary gland (mid-eyebrow): Crystal Palace -- Cavity of the Spirit

Jade Pillow (Yui-Gen -- cranial pump)

Throat center (Hsuan-Chi)

C-7 point (Ta-Chiu))

Thymus Gland and Heart (Shan-Chung) -- rejuvenation center

Point opposite the heart (Gia-Pe)

Solar plexus (Chung-Wen)

T-11 point (Chi-Chung) adrenal gland center

Navel (Chi-Chung)

Sea of Chi (Dan Tien)

Kidney point (Ming-Men) Door of Life

Ovarian Palace / Sperm Palace

Extra 31 (He ding)

Sacral pump Coccyx (Chang-Chiang)

Wei-chung BL-40 extra spirit energy is stored here

Perineum (Hui-Yin) Gate of Death and Life

GOVERNOR CHANNEL

K-1 point (Yung-Chuan) – Bubbling Spring

213

## Opening of the Small Circulation

Basically, the small circulation refers to the practice of regulating and increasing the flow of one's internal energy throughout the conception and governing channels. This increase in energy throughout the body has been known for centuries to promote health and longevity. Beginning meditation training can be started by practicing breathing deeply from the diaphragm or Abdominal Breathing. The Small Circulation can be the next stage of meditation training. Eventually, one can practice the Grand Circulation Meditation, which circulates Qi everywhere in the body. The Grand Circulation, Big Circle or Big Circulation refers to the energy flow through the Twelve Primary Qi channels or meridians. Qigong is interrelated to the energy meridians. When consistent practice reaches a certain level, the individual can feel the Qi and blood flow through the meridians. The paths of the meridians must be some-what familiar while practicing Qigong so as to promote Qi to move along them.

Qigong is one way of strengthening the human body, preventing diseases and prolonging life. It includes two aspects. One being, self-training by performing postures of the human body, regulation of respiration, relaxation of the mind and body, and concentration of one's mind. This aspect is to regulate and strengthen the physical functions of the practitioner's own body. The second aspect is more advanced in that the Qigong specialist can send out their Qi externally to particular areas of another person in order to treat or prevent illness.

Visualize holding a weightless ball between your palms and chest, another within the pelvis. After conforming to the above body alignments, inhale while focusing just below the navel and following your center line between the legs and up the back, over the head and to the spot between the nose & upper lip. Exhale as following your awareness back to just below the navel.

---

Illness and diseases such as addiction, mental health issues, heart disease, diabetes, and mental health issues have all been linked to stress and tension. Meditation and mindfulness-based methods of relaxation have shown potential in bringing about the relaxation response, helping reduce anxiety and enhance well-being. The relaxation response is the term used for the body's physiological response to relieving stress, where respiration and blood pressure is lowered to counter the "fight or flight" response, thereby activating the body's parasympathetic nervous system (Goldsby, et al 2017).

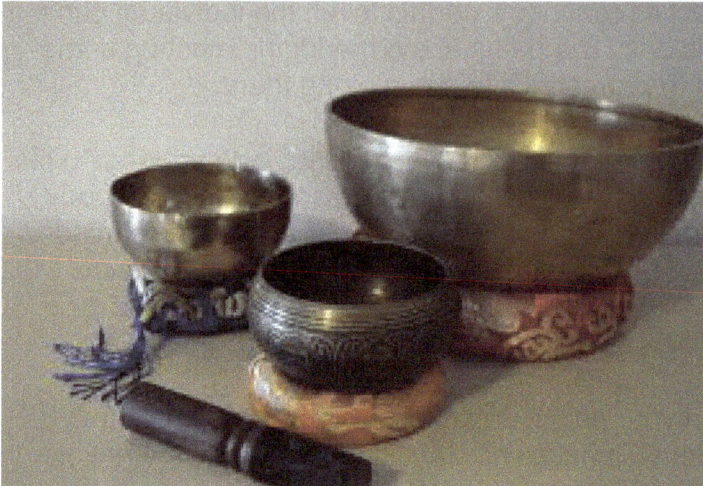

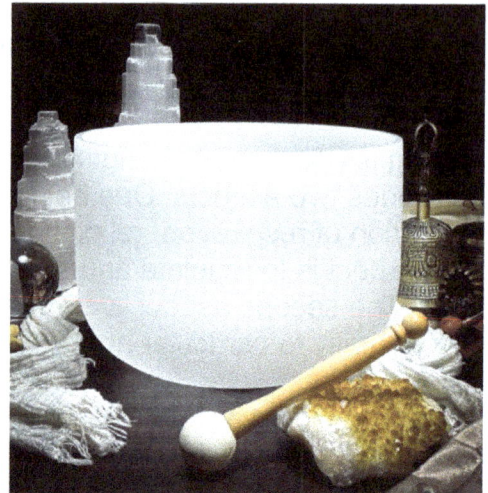

Tibetan or Himalayan singing bowls and other ancient instruments used for religious and spiritual ceremonies have been in practice for a very long time. Use goes back thousands of years, with origins in China and Mongolia. Tibetan Buddhist monasteries used the bowls in this manner to keep time or to signal the end of a meditation (Pikörn 2021). Cultures including native peoples, throughout the world have been using sound for healing for thousands of years. The didgeridoo is an instrument used by Australian aboriginal tribes for over 40,000 years, as a sound healing instrument. (Goldsby, et al 2017).
https://youtu.be/Q2CEtSdVHIU

Contemporary music therapy has been known to benefit suffers of various health conditions, including mental illness and pain. Meditation has long been known to also offer improved health and well-being with modern studies indicating that meditation is effective in managing many ailments. such as anxiety, depression, and pain issues (Stanhope & Weinstein (2020). How singing bowls produces health benefits is ambiguous. While sound bowls can help some people to relax and feel better, more research needs to be done to show how they may be able to target the same regions of the mind that meditation does (Pikörn 2021).

A singing bowl or standing bell are mostly crystal or metal alloy bowls where, by rubbing a mallet around the bowl's outer rim and edges produce sounds. Singing bowls and sometimes gongs surround the user with tones that offer the goal of relaxation by decreasing stress, anxiety, and depression. These sounds offer an escape from the everyday incessant inner dialogue or chatter of thoughts within one's mind. Singing bowl techniques can be very mind engaging, similarly to meditation practices and yoga, and are often practiced in tandem (Pikörn 2021).

Alfred A. Tomatis, a 20th-century French otolaryngologist (one who studies diseases of the ear and throat) offered the thought that music can influence brain waves. Don Campbell's 1997 book, The Mozart Effect, focused on how music could make one smarter and increase concentration (Pikörn 2021).

The Influence of sound on the human mind and consequently the physical body, has been theorized that sound bowls can help calm the mind, by mimicking the brain's electrical impulses, also referred to as "entraining". Here, sound vibrations can "re-tune" the wave patterns of one's mind, in this case Theta brain waves, similar to the vibrations that occur while in states of deep relaxation or concentration. Theta patterns resonate at 4-8 Hertz, occurring also during REM sleep, states of creativity, and during meditation. Studies report the theory that music can indeed change the brain's bio-electrical oscillations. However, this effect is most evident in the range of alpha (8-13 Hertz) and beta (13 Hertz or greater) frequencies. From listening to singing bowls, one can guide their mind towards theta brain wave activity (Pikörn 2021).

A study published in 2017, explored the benefits of using singing bowls along with meditation, using data from a sample of 62 individuals participating. The ages were from 21-77 years old with a mean age 49.7 years. 9 were males and 53 females. The study was held at 3 locations in southern California at The Seaside Center for Spiritual Living in Encinitas, The Chopra Center for Wellbeing in Carlsbad, and the California Institute for Human Science (CIHS) in Encinitas (Goldsby, et al 2017). From my own personal knowledge, I know this particular area of the US to be a hub for meditation and other alternative medicine practices. So, it really didn't surprise me that the results would show that these particular methods yielded positive health benefits. People in the 20-39 age group reported the largest change in a reduction in their tension. However, the study did not specify what type of tension they were experiencing to begin with such as mental, muscular, or otherwise. Those in the 40-59 age group, reported the most noticeable effects from the meditation, with a decrease or even elimination of physical pain before and after the meditation (Goldsby, et al 2017).

It is not hard to find and purchase singing bowls as they are widely available online and elsewhere, costing as little as $20 per bowl and as high as thousands of dollars on the higher end for complete sets of various sizes and compositions. Also available are bowls that will produce different notes and different frequencies. In particular the 432 Hertz range is thought to be more desirable in achieving the desired results of the entraining the theta brain waves. Some avid practitioners of singing bowl meditations prefer usage of the bowls or recorded sounds that are tuned to 432 Hertz. There is also some speculation that listening to music or sounds that have a frequency of 432 Hertz is thought to encourage a positive shift in consciousness, providing the listener with a greater sense of peace. Meditation practitioners seem to favor this music as well. A frequency of 432 Hertz is thought to be the tone of nature, assisting the listener to become more calm, peaceful, and creative. Benefits thought to come from exposure to sounds with the 432 Hertz frequency include release of stress and tension from the body, induction of healing during and after surgeries and the release of endorphins and serotonin (Bawah Reserve 2020).

| Energy Center | Location | Element | Issues | Right | Color | Note |
|---|---|---|---|---|---|---|
| 1st Root | Base of spine | Earth | Physical needs | To have | Red | C |
| 2nd Sacral | Lower abdomen | Water | Sexuality, emotions | To feel | Orange | D |
| 3rd Solar Plexus | Solar plexus | Fire | Power, vitality | To act | Yellow | E |
| 4th Heart | Heart | Air | Love | To love | Green | F |
| 5th Throat | Throat | Sound | Communication | To speak | Blue | G |
| 6th Third Eye | Brow | Light | Intuition | To see | Indigo | A |
| 7th Crown | Top of Head | Thought | Understanding | To know | Violet | B |

It may be that a small group of people have a strong dislike to the sounds made from singing bowls, due to the sounds increasing their self-reported depressions and anxiety. This leads to the possibility that the sound bowls themselves have no special powers of relaxation in and of themselves (Pikörn 2021).

I have studied various methods of using sound with meditation quite a bit over the years and have observed how particular sounds in our daily life, like traffic, thunder, loud music from various genres, yelling, etc. can cause damage to the nervous system. This can happen at the moment or over time, potentially causing even more damage. Consequently, I think the bowls are but another tool to hack the human nervous system to be in a more relaxed state of homeostasis from the parasympathetic nervous system. Any healthcare method that is relatively inexpensive, exhibits no negative side-effects, can easily be obtained by most people, and can offer the user some level of health benefits, is worth further scrutiny and usage by those in particular needing a reduction in their stress levels.

# Glossary

**Abdominal breathing** – effective, diaphragmatic breathing that fills your lungs fully, reaches all the way down to your abdomen, slows your breathing rate, and helps you relax.

Abdominal Movement in Breathing

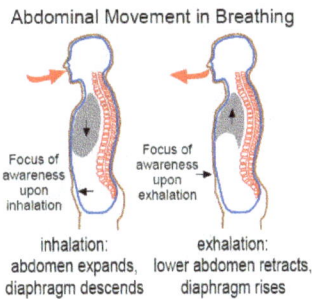

Focus of awareness upon inhalation

Focus of awareness upon exhalation

inhalation: abdomen expands, diaphragm descends

exhalation: lower abdomen retracts, diaphragm rises

**Bagua** (or Pa Kua) / 8-trigrams - eight symbols used in Daoist philosophy to represent the fundamental principles of reality, seen as a range of eight interrelated concepts. Each consists of three lines, each line either "broken" or "unbroken," respectively representing yin or yang.

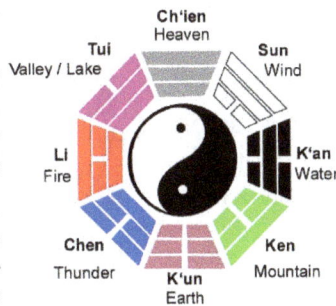

Ch'ien Heaven
Tui Valley / Lake
Sun Wind
Li Fire
K'an Water
Chen Thunder
K'un Earth
Ken Mountain

**The Brass Basin** – sits within the lower abdomen, touching at the navel in the front, between L2 & L3 vertebrae in the back and the perineum at the base.

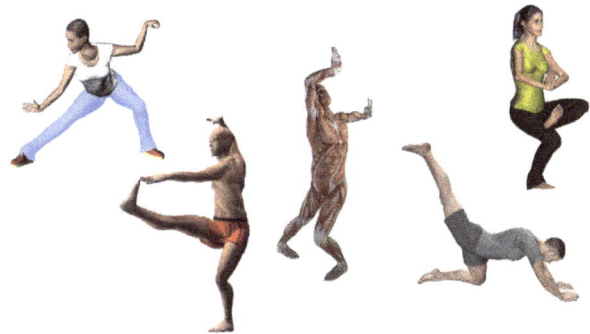

Mingmen-GV4 L2-L3, Gate of Life Kidney Point

Qihai-CV6 Sea of Qi, Navel Point, Spleen

Hui Yin-CV1 Meeting of Yin Gate of Life and Death Perineum

**Bubbling Well** - an energetic point located in the sole of the foot, slightly in front of the arch between the 2nd and 3rd toe. In the meridian system it is the same as the Kidney 1 point.

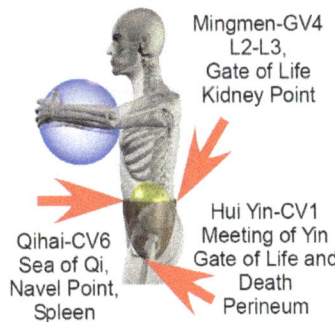

Kidney-1

**Dan Tian** - 3 energy centers Lower Dan Tian (1 of 3) - also known as the "sea of qi," is positioned below and behind the naval encompassing your lower bowl and is closely related to jing (or physical essence).

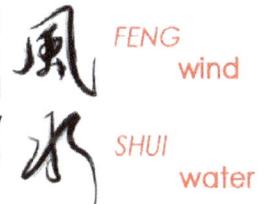

Shen-Spirit Upper Dantian (Field of Light)

Qi-Energy Middle Dantian (Field of Vibration)

Jing-Essence Lower Dantian (Field of Heat)

**Daoyin, DaoYi, Daoist Yoga, Qigong** – all names for energy exercises, with specific postures, little or no physical body movement and mindful regulated breathing patterns.

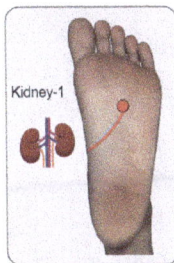

**Feng Shui** – translated into 'wind and water'; it is a Chinese philosophical system that teaches how to balance the energies in any given space.

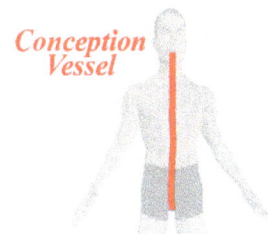

FENG wind

SHUI water

**Conception Vessel** (Ren Mai) – flows up the midline of the front of the body and governs all of the yin channels. The Conception Vessel is connected to the Thrusting and Yin Linking vessels.

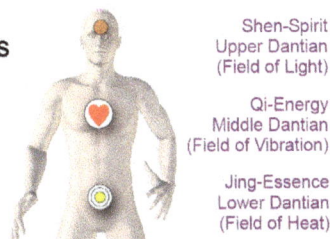

Conception Vessel

**Governing Vessel** (Du Mai) - flows up the midline of the back and governs all the Yang channels.

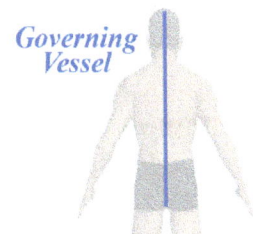

Governing Vessel

**General Yu Fei** – creator of the 8 Pieces of Brocade set.

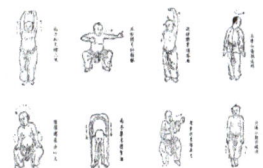

**Controlling Cycle** – the controlling or regulating sequence of the 5 element cycle. Wood controls Earth; Earth controls Water; Water controls Fire; Fire controls Metal; Metal controls Wood

**Generating Cycle** – the creative sequence of the 5 element cycle. Wood generates Fire; Fire generates Earth; Earth generates Metal; Metal generates Water; Water generates Wood.

**Horary Cycle -** 24 Hour Qi Flow Though the Meridians; This cycle is known as the Horary cycle or the Circadian Clock. As Qi (energy) makes its way through the meridians, each meridian in turn with its associated organ, has a two-hour period during which it is at maximum energy.

**Jing Well** - The Jing (Well) points are 1 of 5 of The Five Element Points (shu) of the 12 energy meridians. They are located on the fingers and toes of the four extremities. These points are thought to be where the Qi of the meridians emerges and begins moving towards the trunk of the body. These are of upmost importance in that these points can help restore balance within the energy flow throughout the human body.

**Meridians** - a meridian is an 'energy highway' in the human body. There are 12 meridians and each is paired with an organ. Qi energy flows through these meridians or energy highways.

**Qigong** - or Chi Kung, is breathing exercises, with little or no body movement, that can adjust the brain waves to the Alpha state. When the mind is relaxed, the body chemistry changes and promotes natural healing.

**San Jiao** (Triple Burner/Heater) – is a meridian line that regulates respiration, digestion and elimination. It is responsible for the movement and transformation of various solids and fluids throughout the system, as well as for the production and circulation of nourishing and protective energy.

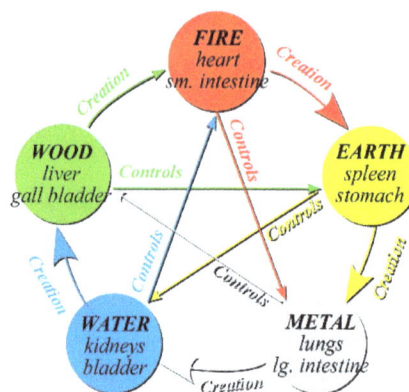

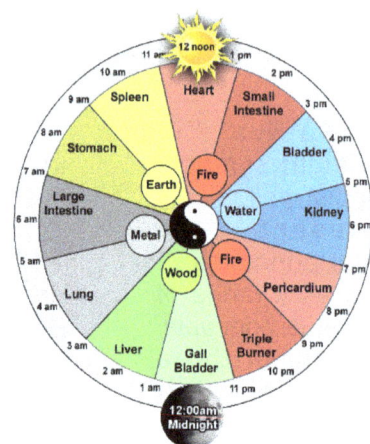

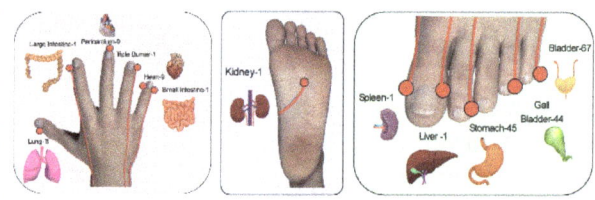

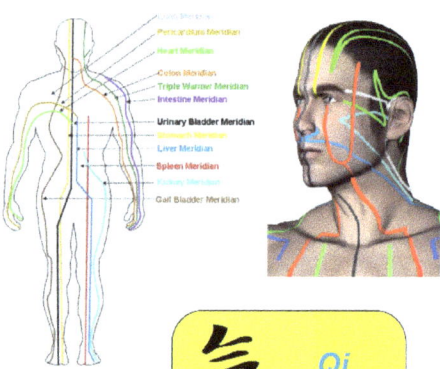

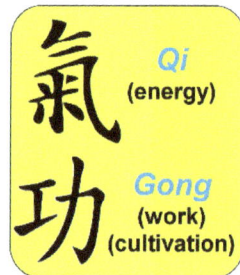

| Upper Burner | WEI QI |
| Middle Burner | YING QI |
| Lower Burner | YUAN QI |

219

**Nine Gates** - the energy gates in your body are major relay stations where the strength of your Qi are regulated. These gates are located at joints or, more precisely, in the actual space between the bones of a joint. The nine gates are located at the shoulder, elbow and wrists, hip, knee and ankles, and along the cervical, the thoracic, and the lumbar spine.

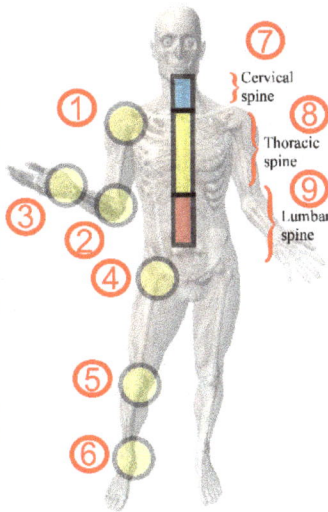

**Seven Energy Centers** – also known as chakras, are energy points in the subtle body that start at the base of the spinal column, continue through the sacral, solar plexus, heart, throat, eyebrow and end in the midst of the head vertex at the crown.

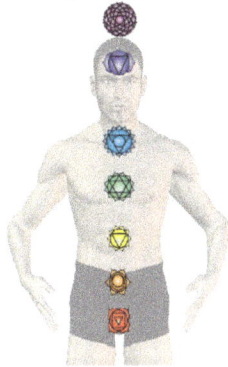

**Three Treasures** – Jing, Qi & Shen

**Jing** – (essence) the physical, yin and most dense of the Three Treasures. Think of Jing as a candle, specifically the quality and quantity of the wax.

**Qi,** chi or ki - (energy/breath) the energetic, vital force within all living things and it the most refined Treasure. Think of Qi as the burning flame of the candle.

**Shen** – (consciousness or spirit, is the most subtle of the Three Treasures and is the vitality behind Jing and Qi. Think of Shen as the light or illumination produced from the flame.

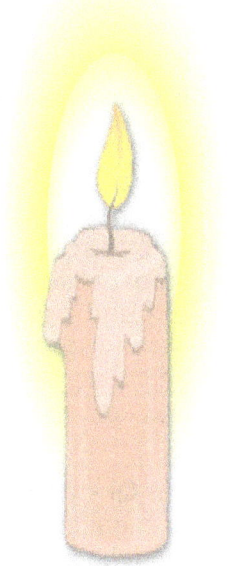

**Six Healing Sounds** – auditory sounds used for clearing internal (yin) organs and other tissues of stagnant Qi.

| Metal - Hissss | Water - Chuuu | Wood - Shiiiii | Fire - Haaaa | Earth - Hoooo | 6th Qi - Heeee |
|---|---|---|---|---|---|
| Lungs Lg. Intestine | Kidneys Bladder | Liver Gall Bladder | Heart Sm. Intestine | Spleen Stomach | Pericardium Triple Burner |

**The 3 Hearts** – Heart, abdomen, calves: The first heart is the heart in your chest for the oxygenation of the blood. Lower abdominal breathing is considered the second heart for circulation of fluid, Qi and digestion. The third heart is the calf muscles for re-circulation of the blood.

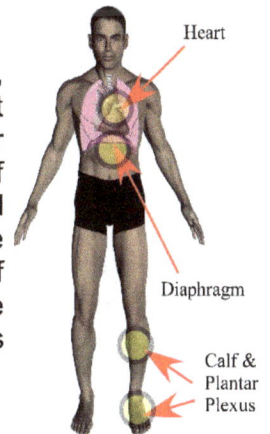

**Small Circuit** – the linking two energy pathways that run along the midline of the body into a cycling loop. The "fire pathway", Du Mai (Governing Vessel), extends up the back and the other, Ren Mai (Conception Vessel), down the front of the body.

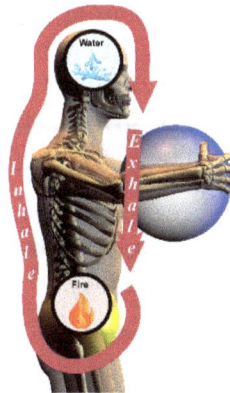

**Vessels** – there are 8 extraordinary vessels that function as reservoirs of Qi for the Twelve Regular Meridians.

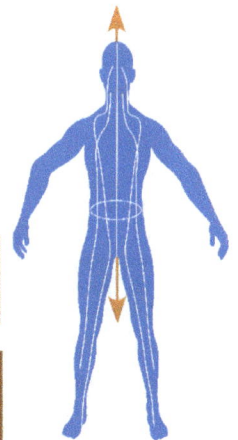

| Conception Thrusting Yin Linking Yin Heel | 4 Yin Vessels |
|---|---|
| Governing Belt Yang Linking Yang Heel | 4 Yang Vessels |

**Taoism** - (sometimes Daoism) is a philosophical or ethical tradition of Chinese origin, or faith of Chinese exemplification, that emphasizes living in harmony with the Tao (or Dao). The term Tao means "way", "path", or the "principle".

220

**The Void (Supreme Mystery)**

**Wuji** – ultimate stillness, the beginning of creation.

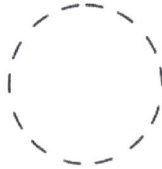

**Yang Qi** - yang refers to aspects or manifestations of Qi that are relatively positive: Also - immaterial, amorphous, expanding, hollow, light, ascending, hot, dry, warming, bright, aggressive, masculine and active.

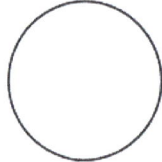

**Yin Qi** - yin refers to aspects or manifestations of Qi that are relatively negative: Also - material, substantial, condensing, solid, heavy, descending, cold, moist, cooling, dark, female, passive and quiescent.

**Taijitu** -The term taijitu in modern Chinese is commonly used to mean the simple "divided circle" form (), but it may refer to any of several schematic diagrams that contain at least one circle with an inner pattern of symmetry representing yin and yang.

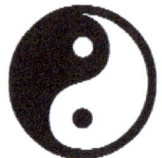

**Yi** – intellect, manifests as spirit-infused intelligence and understanding.

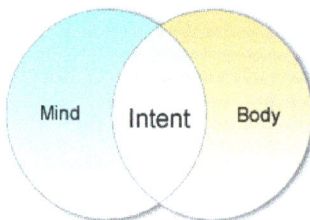

Mind    Intent    Body

**Baihui point** - Governing Vessel 20 (GV 20). Sits on the crown of the head.

**Jade Pillow** – located at the top of the cervical vertebrae (C1).

**Great Hammer** – located on the midline at the base of the neck, between seventh cervical vertebra and first thoracic vertebra.

**Mingmen point** – Conception Vessel 6 (CV6), the 'Sea of Qi' located on the lower abdomen.

**Qihai point** – Conception Vessel 6 (CV6), the 'Sea of Qi' located on the lower abdomen.

**Hui Yin point** – Conception Vessel 1 (CV1), also known as the base chakra, is located between the genitals and the anus; the part of the body called the perineum.

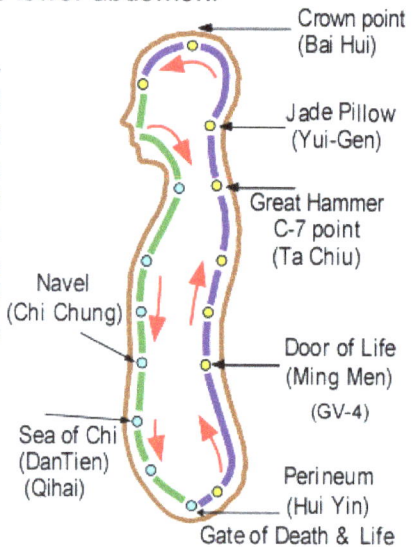

Crown point (Bai Hui)
Jade Pillow (Yui-Gen)
Great Hammer C-7 point (Ta Chiu)
Door of Life (Ming Men) (GV-4)
Navel (Chi Chung)
Sea of Chi (DanTien) (Qihai)
Perineum (Hui Yin)
Gate of Death & Life

**Wu Xing or 5 Elements** -
The 5 Element theory is a major component of thought within Traditional Chinese Medicine (TCM). Each element represents natural aspects within our world. Natural cycles and interrelationships between these elements, is the basis for this theory. These elements have corresponding relationships within our environment as well as within our own being.

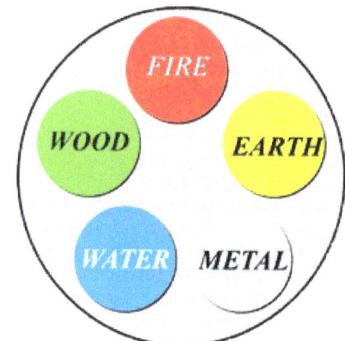

FIRE
WOOD    EARTH
WATER    METAL

**Zang-Fu organs** – solid, yin organs are Zang – yang and hollow organs are Fu.

| 5 Yin Organs | Liver, Heart, Spleen, Lungs, Kidneys |
|---|---|

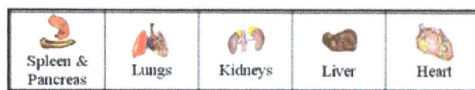

| | Spleen & Pancreas | Lungs | Kidneys | Liver | Heart |
|---|---|---|---|---|---|

| 5 Yang Organs | Gall Bladder, Small Intestine, Stomach, Large Intestine, Bladder |
|---|---|

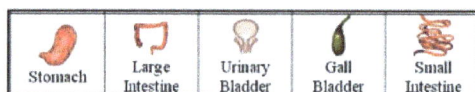

| | Stomach | Large Intestine | Urinary Bladder | Gall Bladder | Small Intestine |
|---|---|---|---|---|---|

221

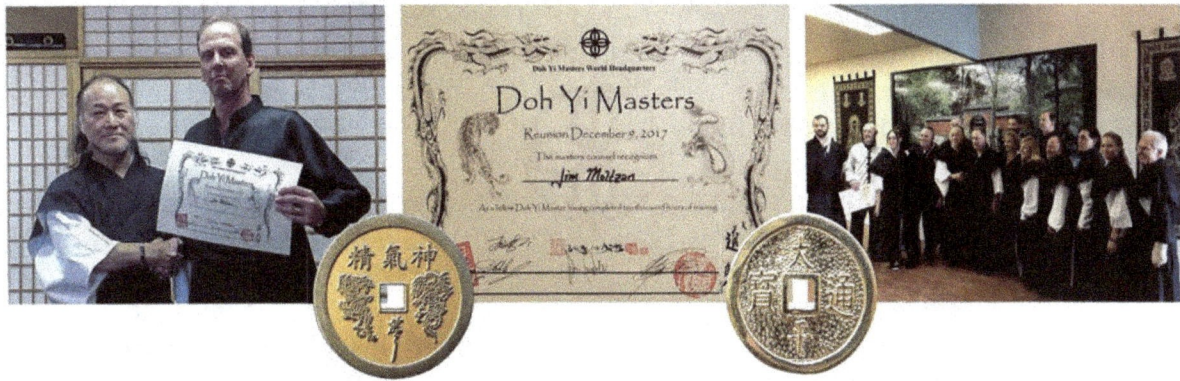

## About the Instructor, Author & Artist - Jim Moltzan

My fitness training started at the age of 16 and has continued for almost 45 years. During that time, I attended high school, then college, and worked 2 jobs all while pursuing further training in martial arts and other fitness methods. Many years ago, I started up an additional business to help finance my next goal of owning my own school. I moved to Florida from the Midwest to make this goal a reality. Having owned two wellness and martial arts schools, I have surpassed what I once believed to be my potential. At this stage in my life, I have chosen not to open any more schools, as I found the business aspects took too much focus away from my true passion: training and teaching others.

Beyond my professional endeavors, I am also a husband and father of two grown children. I believe that we must be prepared to work hard mentally, physically and financially to earn our good health and well-being. Not only for ourselves but for our families as well. Good health always comes at a cost whether in time, effort, cost, sacrifice or some combination of the previous.

I returned to college in my later 50's, to pursue my BS in Holistic Health (wellness and alternative medicine). My degree program covered many wide-ranging topics such as anatomy and physiology, meditation, massage, nutrition, herbology, chemistry, biology, history and basis of various medical modalities such as allopathic, Traditional Chinese Medicine, Ayurveda/yoga, naturopathy, chiropractic, and complimentary alternative methods. I also studied religion, mythology of the world, stress relief/management as well as sociology, psychology (human behavior) and cultural issues associated with better health and wellness.

Most of the movements I teach and write about originate from Chinese martial arts. The Qigong (breathing work) is from Chinese Kung Fu and the Korean Dong Han medical Qigong lineage. I have also gained much knowledge of Traditional Chinese Medicine (TCM) from many TCM practitioners, martial arts masters, teachers and peers. This includes many techniques and practices of acupressure (reflexology, auricular, Jing Well, etc.), acupuncture, moxibustion as well as preparation of some herbal remedies and extracts for conditioning and injuries. I have been studying for over 20 years with Zen Wellness, learning medical Qigong as well as other Eastern methods of fitness, philosophy and self-cultivation. I have been recognized as a "Gold Coin" master instructor having trained and taught others for at least 10000 hours or roughly over 35 years. The core fitness movements are from Kung Fu and its forms in Tai Chi, Baguazhang, Dao Yin and Ship Pal Gi (Korean Kung Fu and weapons training). Each martial art has mental, physical and spiritual aspects that can complement and enhance one another. The more ways that you can move your body and engage your mind, the better it is for your overall health.

Physical health, mental well-being and the relationships within our lives; are these the most cherished aspects of our existence? Yet, how much effort do we put towards improving these areas on a daily basis?

Many have used martial arts and other mind-body methods of training as methods of learning to see one's character as others see them. I feel that I can offer the priceless qualities of truth, honor and integrity with my instruction. You must seek the right teacher for you, because in time a student can become similar to their teacher. Through the training that I have experienced and offer to others, an individual can understand and hopefully reach their full potential.

By developing self-discipline to continuously execute and perfect sets of movements, an individual can start to understand not only how they work physically but also mentally and emotionally. You can find your strengths and your weaknesses and improve them both. Through disciplined training, one not only enhances physical abilities but also cultivates mental resilience, allowing them to achieve their fullest potential in all areas of life.

I have co-authored a book, produced numerous other books and journals, graphic charts and study guides related to the mind and body connection and how it relates to martial arts, fitness, and self-improvement. A few hundred of my classes and lectures are viewable on YouTube.com.

## Lineage

o   Recognized as a 1000 and 10,000-hour student and teacher

o   Earned gold coins through the Doh Yi Masters and Zen Wellness program

o   Earned a 5th degree in Korean Kung Fu through the Dong Han lineage

## Education

Bachelor of Science in Holistic Medicine - Vermont State University

# Books Available Through Amazon

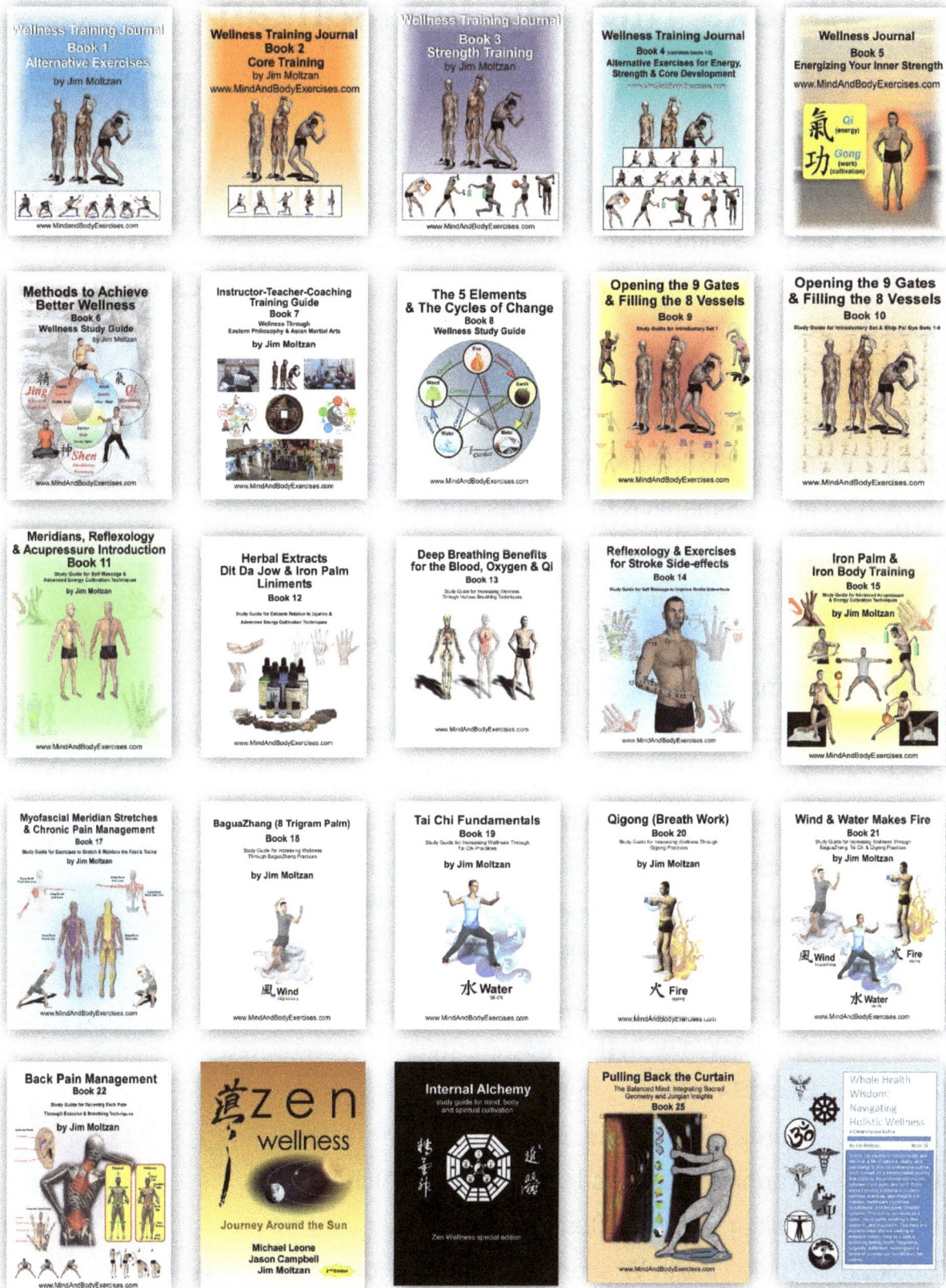

**Wellness Training Journal Book 1 Alternative Exercises** by Jim Moltzan
www.MindandBodyExercises.com

**Wellness Training Journal Book 2 Core Training** by Jim Moltzan
www.MindAndBodyExercises.com

**Wellness Training Journal Book 3 Strength Training** by Jim Moltzan
www.MindandBodyExercises.com

**Wellness Training Journal Book 4** Alternative Exercises for Energy, Strength & Core Development
www.MindAndBodyExercises.com

**Wellness Journal Book 5 Energizing Your Inner Strength**
www.MindAndBodyExercises.com
Qi (energy) Gong (work) (cultivation)

**Methods to Achieve Better Wellness Book 6 Wellness Study Guide** by Jim Moltzan
Jing Qi Shen
www.MindAndBodyExercises.com

**Instructor-Teacher-Coaching Training Guide Book 7** Wellness Through Eastern Philosophy & Asian Martial Arts by Jim Moltzan
www.MindAndBodyExercises.com

**The 5 Elements & The Cycles of Change Book 8 Wellness Study Guide**
www.MindAndBodyExercises.com

**Opening the 9 Gates & Filling the 8 Vessels Book 9** Study Guide for Introductory Set 1

**Opening the 9 Gates & Filling the 8 Vessels Book 10** Study Guide for Introductory Set & Ship Pal Gya Sets 1-8

**Meridians, Reflexology & Acupressure Introduction Book 11** Study Guide for Self Massage & Advanced Energy Cultivation Techniques by Jim Moltzan
www.MindAndBodyExercises.com

**Herbal Extracts Dit Da Jow & Iron Palm Liniments Book 12** Study Guide for Extracts Relative to Injuries & Advanced Energy Cultivation Techniques

**Deep Breathing Benefits for the Blood, Oxygen & Qi Book 13** Study Guide for Increasing Wellness Through Various Breathing Techniques
www.MindAndBodyExercises.com

**Reflexology & Exercises for Stroke Side-effects Book 14** Study Guide for Self Massage to Improve Stroke Side-effects

**Iron Palm & Iron Body Training Book 15** Study Guide for Advanced Acupressure & Energy Cultivation Techniques by Jim Moltzan
www.MindAndBodyExercises.com

**Myofascial Meridian Stretches & Chronic Pain Management Book 17** Study Guide for Exercises to Stretch & Maintain the Fascia Trains by Jim Moltzan
www.MindAndBodyExercises.com

**BaguaZhang (8 Trigram Palm) Book 18** Study Guide for Increasing Wellness Through BaguaZhang Practices by Jim Moltzan
Wind
www.MindAndBodyExercises.com

**Tai Chi Fundamentals Book 19** Study Guide for Increasing Wellness Through Tai Chi Practices by Jim Moltzan
Water
www.MindAndBodyExercises.com

**Qigong (Breath Work) Book 20** Study Guide for Increasing Wellness Through Qigong Practices by Jim Moltzan
Fire
www.MindAndBodyExercises.com

**Wind & Water Makes Fire Book 21** Study Guide for Increasing Wellness Through BaguaZhang, Tai Chi & Qigong Practices by Jim Moltzan
Wind Fire Water
www.MindAndBodyExercises.com

**Back Pain Management Book 22** Study Guide for Relieving Back Pain Through Exercise & Breathing Techniques by Jim Moltzan
www.MindAndBodyExercises.com

**zen wellness** Journey Around the Sun
Michael Leone Jason Campbell Jim Moltzan
2nd Edition

**Internal Alchemy** study guide for mind, body and spiritual cultivation
Zen Wellness special edition

**Pulling Back the Curtain** The Integration of Sacred Geometry and Jungian Insights **Book 25**
www.MindAndBodyExercises.com

**Whole Health Wisdom: Navigating Holistic Wellness** A Comprehensive Guide to
by Jim Moltzan

# Books Titles by Jim Moltzan

**On Amazon**

Book 1 - Alternative Exercises

Book 2 - Core Training

Book 3 - Strength Training

Book 4 - Combo of 1-3

Book 5 - Energizing Your Inner Strength

Book 6 - Methods to Achieve Better Wellness

Book 7 - Coaching & Instructor Training Guide

Book 8 - The 5 Elements & the Cycles of Change

Book 9 - Opening the 9 Gates & Filling 8 Vessels - Intro Set 1

Book 10 - Opening the 9 Gates & Filling 8 Vessels-sets 1 to 8

Book 11 - Meridians, Reflexology & Acupressure

Book 12 - Herbal Extracts, Dit Da Jow & Iron Palm Liniments

Book 13 - Deep Breathing Benefits for the Blood, Oxygen & Qi

Book 14 - Reflexology for Stroke Side Effects:

Book 15 - Iron Body & Iron Palm

Book 17 - Fascial Train Stretches & Chronic Pain Management

Book 18 - BaguaZhang

Book 19 - Tai Chi Fundamentals

Book 20 - Qigong (breath-work)

Book 21 - Wind & Water Make Fire

Book 22 - Back Pain Management

Book 23 - Journey Around the Sun-2nd Edition

Book 24 - Graphic Reference Book - Internal Alchemy

Book 25 – Pulling Back the Curtain

Book 26 - Whole Health Wisdom: Navigating Holistic Wellness

# Other Products

## Laminated Charts 8.5" x 11" or 11" x 17" - over 200 various graphics (check the website)

### Qigong - Chi Kung
SKU: ChiKung

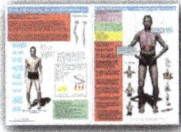

The human body is made up of bones, muscles, and organs amongst other components. Veins, arteries and capillaries carry blood and nutrients throughout to all of the systems and components. Additionally, 12 major energy medians carry the body's energy, "life force" also known as "chi". Ones chi is stored in the lower Dan Tien. Daily emotional imbalances accumulate tension and stress gradually affecting all of the body's systems. Each discomfort, nuisance, irritation or grudge continues to tighten and squeeze the flow of the life force. This is where "dis-ease" claims its foothold.

### Strengthen Your Back (set #1)
SKU: StrengthenYourBack1

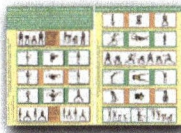

Good health of the lower back starts with good posture. The following set of exercises develop strength and flexibility which improve posture. Strength in the back, hips and abdominals provide a strong cage that houses the internal organs. Flexibility in these areas helps to maintain good blood circulation to the organs and lower body. Lengthening of the spine while exercising reduces stress and tension on the nervous system.

### Broadsword 1-10
SKU: Broadsword

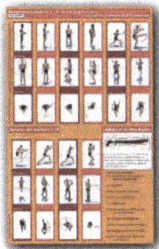

Broadsword training develops the body, mind and spirit well beyond that which can gained from empty hand training alone. The Broadsword has many different sets to be mastered utilizing quick, fluid and precise movements.

### Ship Pal Gye set 7 (Kung Fu stance training)
SKU: ShipPalGye7

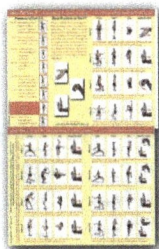

SHIP PAL GYE or Ship Par Gay, is a Korean version of Chinese Shaolin Lohan Qigong, meaning "18 chi movements" or what were supposedly the original 18 drills that Bodhidharma introduced to the Shaolin monks. It is reputed to be the basis for the Shaolin Kung Fu, which in turn, greatly influenced the developments of all branches of Asian fighting arts.

### Noble Stances
SKU: NobleStances

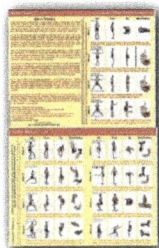

Noble stances are a combination of various stances from different styles of Chinese martial arts. Stances, in this case, meaning correct placement of the feet, knees, hips, and arm positions relative to ones center of gravity. Executing static positions and holding the particular body positions for anyway from a few seconds to several minutes reaps many benefits foremost being able to cultivate a strong and healthy core.

# Contacts

For more information regarding charts, products, classes and instruction:

www.MindAndBodyExercises.com
info@MindAndBodyExercises.com

www.youtube.com/c/MindandBodyExercises
www.MindAndBodyExercises.wordpress.com

407-234-0119

Social Media:

Facebook:      MindAndBodyExercises
Instagram:     MindAndBodyExercises
Twitter:       MindAndBodyExercise

Jim Moltzan - Mind and Body Exercises
522 Hunt Club Blvd. #305
Apopka, FL 32703

**Website**

**Blog**

**YouTube
Channel**